CONCORDIA UNIVERSITY

RJ503.C66   C001 V
TEXTBOOK OF ADOLESCENT PSYCHOPATHOL

3 4211 000096737

WITHDRAWN

DATE DUE

APR 0 4 2002		

DEMCO 38-297

D1161108

Textbook of
Adolescent
Psychopathology
and Treatment

Textbook of Adolescent Psychopathology and Treatment

By

ADRIAN D. COPELAND, M.S., M.D.

Clinical Associate Professor
Chief of Adolescent Psychiatric Services
Department of Psychiatry and Human Behavior
Thomas Jefferson University School of Medicine
Philadelphia, Pennsylvania

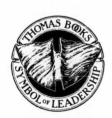

KLINCK MEMORIAL LIBRARY
Concordia Teachers College
River Forest, Illinois 60305

CHARLES C THOMAS • PUBLISHER
Springfield • Illinois • U.S.A.

Published and Distributed Throughout the World by
CHARLES C THOMAS • PUBLISHER
Bannerstone House
301-327 East Lawrence Avenue, Springfield, Illinois, U.S.A.

This book is protected by copyright. No part of it
may be reproduced in any manner without written
permission from the publisher.

©*1974, by* CHARLES C THOMAS • PUBLISHER
ISBN 0-398-03114-2 (cloth)
ISBN 0-398-03115-0 (paper)
Library of Congress Catalog Card Number: 73-23012

*With THOMAS BOOKS careful attention is given to all details of
manufacturing and design. It is the Publisher's desire to present books that are
satisfactory as to their physical qualities and artistic possibilities and
appropriate for their particular use. THOMAS BOOKS will be true to those
laws of quality that assure a good name and good will.*

Printed in the United States of America
N-10

Library of Congress Cataloging in Publication Data

Copeland, Adrian D

Library of Congress Cataloging in Publication Data

Copeland, Adrian D
    Textbook of adolescent psychopathology and treatment.

    1. Adolescent psychiatry. I. Title.
[DNLM: 1. Affective disturbances–In adolescence.
2. Affective disturbances–Therapy. WS462 C782t 1974]
RJ503.C66   618.9'28'9   73-23012
ISBN 0-398-03114-2
ISBN 0-398-03115-0 (pkb.)

The purchase of this material was 124547
made possible by a grant from
THE AID ASSOCIATION FOR LUTHERANS

This book is dedicated to my family: to my parents; to my wife, Elise, for her technical help and good ideas; and to Loren, Ron, Graham and Dan for teaching me so much about adolescence.

CONTENTS

Textbook of
Adolescent
Psychopathology
and Treatment

CHAPTER I

INTRODUCTION

ALTHOUGH much has been written about the emotional problems of adolescence, few textbooks have emerged to date. This paucity alone is reason enough to write such a book, but the urgency of the subject should be considered as well.

Youth constitutes a large and important segment of the population, and there is considerable evidence that it is a group currently under a great deal of stress. While the overall census in mental hospitals is declining, more young people are becoming institutionalized for psychological disorders than ever before. The problem of drug misuse and emotional breakdown is essentially a problem of youth. Gang violence and educational default or "dropping out" are two further illustrations of adolescent stress and breakdown.

There are clear indications of a widespread adolescent stress syndrome identified by gloominess and a preoccupation with disaster. Far from being carefree, many young people today are oriented instead towards the dangers of atomic extinction, overpopulation and world pollution. They have been profoundly influenced by a parlor device, television, which has beamed continuous messages of violence and destruction for as long as this generation can remember. Contemporary life stresses have been considerable, and youths' reaction has been equally profound.

With this backdrop of pessimism concerning the human condition, many adolescents have alienated themselves from the less compelling problems of survival and adaptation, thus reducing their overall stress.

The roots of these pressures are multiple. The contemporary American society has contributed to a great degree. As a technocracy seeking to maintain its position of world primacy, it has placed great educational demands upon its young people. Ever-increasing volumes of technical information must be mastered; educational curriculae must be constantly revised and upgraded to keep pace with this information explosion, and students must face the inevitability of increasingly prolonged periods of academic dependence.

Compensations for assuming these culturally desired burdens, however, are often remote, uncertain or insufficient; witness the periodic economic downturns that produce unemployment even among the ranks of the most highly skilled.

In addition to the culturally induced problems of increasing demands and uncertain rewards, there is also the very serious stress of inadequate emotional and psychological support. Security provided by time-hallowed traditions and values has given way to transition and uncertainty. The primary family unit has been devitalized by divorce and the breakdown of traditional parental roles. The extended family system, which has functioned as an auxiliary support for young people, has been decimated by a national mobility and rootlessness. Organized religion, too, has been torn by the issue of its own relevance, thereby casting further doubt and uncertainty into the lives of young people.

What then is there for youth to rely on? Nothing, except youth itself; and this conviction has been one of its essential unifying and strengthening forces.

Demographically, young people are important and demand to be heard. Their commentary provides much valuable information not only about the problems of society but also about their own problems as well.

As clinicians from the many and varied disciplines that treat the psychological problems of young people, it behooves us to listen to them and try to understand them. For inevitably they will emerge from adolescence into adulthood and, if we do our jobs well, we may contribute to some small degree to their success in establishing a cleaner, saner planetary existence tomorrow.

CHAPTER II

ADOLESCENCE AND NORMALITY

INTRODUCTION

AT a time when clinicians are seeing and treating ever-increasing numbers of young people, it is important to have criteria to determine what constitutes mental health and what constitutes mental illness. Yet the concept of normality, especially as applied to adolescence, is exceedingly imprecise. *Random House Dictionary* lists eight definitions of normality, related to three different disciplines of human endeavor.

In medicine the original use of the term was predicated upon organic factors, and normality was simply the absence of gross tissue pathology or infectious organisms.

Offer and Sabshin (1966) note four possible meanings for the term normality: (1) health; (2) optimal function; (3) statistical averages for certain traits, e.g. intelligence; (4) a temporary equilibrium state, as noted in Hippocrates' balance with nature and Cannon's concept of hemeostasis.

In general terms, then, normality may be related to survival and adaptation.

SOCIOLOGICAL CONSIDERATIONS

From a sociological point of view, "normal" behavior is a reflection of cultural values and is thus relative.

A clinical diagnosis can be an indication of cultural distance and bias, as in the case of the upper middle class white psychiatrist's inappropriate labelling of black ghetto youth as "unsocialized aggressive" or "group delinquent" (Brickman).

Subcultural value differences must also be considered when

clinicians espousing "establishment" standards are asked to evaluate the behavior of adherents of a youth culture. A different point of view does not necessarily make a case for the diagnosis of psychopathology (Beckett, Lorande, Mead).

Hypotheses Relating Societal Transition and Normality

In general, standards of normality tend to change as the needs and sociodynamics of a culture change. In such times of transition, the labelling of a behavior as "normal" or "abnormal" is difficult to justify. Pressures to alter the norms of society may come from without, as illustrated in the impact of American occupation forces upon Japan after World War II. Pressures may also come from within, as noted in the impact of youth upon the whole matrix of the contemporary American society (Mead). Many traditional norms are thus altered. Behavior considered abnormal before is less recognized as pathological today, e.g. running away, premarital intercourse, and the use of drugs.

Normality, from a cultural standpoint, implies two modes of adaptation: absolute (dealing with problems of physical survival) and relative (dealing with the individual's relation to the culture). Parameters of cultural normality are role, function, attitudes, and behavior. Judgments about normality are made in terms of the individual's degree of compliance to the standards set for these parameters. Individual response ranges between minimally acceptable and optimal; failure to meet the minimal standards evokes the judgment "abnormal."

Such judgments pertain only where cultural values and roles are clear, stable and universally accepted. Conversely, cultures in transition render pronouncements about an individual's normality tenuous. Changing gender-roles in contemporary America is an illustration. Whereas the traditional role of the male has been to provide food and shelter and that of the female to provide nesting and nurture, pressures for reversal have shaken these standards radically.

Thus, from a cultural point of view, normality deals with the issue of how members of a society shall achieve optimal adaptation at a particular point in time.

CLINICAL CONSIDERATIONS

To clinically assess the mental health or psychological normality of the adolescent, the clinician must take cognizance of the following factors:

I. His operant value system
II. Psychological characteristics of adolescence
III. His adaptational success
IV. His mental status
V. The experienced clinician's intuitive response.

The Adolescent's Operant Value System

It is essential to establish which value system or subculture a particular adolescent subscribes to before making clinical judgments about his behavior. Farnsworth (1966) cites three such value systems affecting youth: traditional morality, the new morality, and amorality. Other codes no doubt exist and require further investigation and analysis. There is a value system influencing the behavior of black ghetto youth, of Ivy League youth, of Bible belt youth, and youth of different ethnic subcultures. Drug taking as a cultural norm had been noted among Mexican-Americans long before the current drug pandemic.

Psychological Characteristics of Adolescence

'Adolescence is a phase of turmoil and transition producing behavior that would be considered unusual or bizarre at any other period.' Much of this normal abnormality is temporary and not indicative of mental illness, but rather a reaction to a period of developmental stress. Persistence into adulthood, however, would be indicative of true psychopathology.

Adequate understanding of adolescent idiosyncrasies, then, is essential in differentiating true persistant pathological processes from transitional peculiarities.

Characteristics of Adolescent Thinking

Preoccupation with the Self (Redl)

The positive aspect of this preoccupation, referred to by Blos and Jacobson as narcissism, is but one kind of intense involvement with the self at this phase. Frequently coupled with self-love is the intense self-doubt which often produces ideas of omnipotence paired closely with crises of self-confidence.

Preoccupation with Phantasy

This preoccupation is borne of intense drives and feelings that are developing at this time, and phantasy serves as a means of containing these drives and at the same time providing some gratification of them.

Preoccupation with the Need for Self-expression

"Doing your own thing" reflects the need to establish autonomy and freedom from parental supervision and consent. Being unique, then, occupies an important part of adolescent thinking and is more related to the process of separation from the dependent position and establishing a sense of identity than to being outstanding and famous.

Preoccupation with Philosophical Abstractions, Theories and Ideals (Piaget, 1969)

This is the phase of life where one actively ponders such questions as "absolute truth," "ultimate reality," or the riddle of infinity. It is a time for evolving newer and better theories and becoming intoxicated with new discoveries; a time for abject disdain for already delineated ideas that have not worked perfectly. Much of this spirit is inherent in youth's impatience with age and its revolutionary zeal. Adolescence is the time to question, reject and propose new theoretical solutions. Focus on societal ills serves this purpose very well.

Preoccupation with Sexuality

This is manifested by an intense interest in things sexual, whether they be genitals or the secondary sex characteristics such as breasts or hair. It may take a fetishistic form and focus on articles of clothing. As adolescence progresses, sexuality becomes more object-oriented, and initial heterosexual relationships can take the form of "crushes," characterized by intense longing without gratification, or "puppy love," represented by the over-idealization of the love relationship.

Among boys there is usually intense masturbatory activity, while adolescent girls become more sensuous generally, with less differentiated genital focus than boys. Much preening and grooming behavior is notable, and homosexual experimentation is not uncommon. Adolescence, then, is a time of heightened sex drives and gender-specific differences in their manifestation.

Hedonism and/or Asceticism

Hedonism and asceticism may be understood in terms of the young person in relation to his drives, with full pursuit of instinctual gratification evident in the case of hedonism and renunciation of the drives from fear and guilt noted in asceticism. This guilt and fear may be sufficiently severe to produce withdrawal from all object relationships. Asceticism is probably more psychopathological than hedonism.

Conformism

In the midst of the adolescent's struggle to move from the position of dependency to that of individuality and self-reliance, identification with a chosen peer group is a necessary transitional phase. As he shifts his identificational patterns, he takes on the characteristics of that group. His conformism to a new set of standards is the necessary intermediate step towards the evolution of the sense of self. Particular styles of dress and behavior have always been characteristic of the adolescent phase and have always drawn criticism from the adult sector.

Characteristics of Adolescent Affects and Behavior

Heightened Sensitivity (Sklansky)

The adolescent often experiences things with great intensity and strong passions, sometimes overreacting. Most anything can be a cause célèbre. He is indifferent to very little.

Mood Swings

Joy and sadness can occur suddenly and almost simultaneously at this phase. When similar shifts of affect are noted in the adult, it may be considered pathological.

Propensity to "Act Out"

This may be defined simply as the tendency to cause trouble for oneself or for others by virtue of impulsive behavior which is a reflection of unconscious conflicts and problems (Sklansky). Carried to an extreme it may take the form of rebelliousness, delinquency, or even more organized insurrectionist behavior (Blos, 1962).

Inhibition of Behavior

This may occur transitorily, coupled with withdrawal (Sklansky). It may be associated with asceticism. (See guilt disturbance, Ch. II)

Developmental Tasks and Adaptational Success

¹ The capacity to adapt successfully to one's environment is considered one of the hallmarks of normality, and this is especially true in the adolescent phase, where the tasks of adaptation are numerous and crucial.¹ The following parameters of successful adaptation are derived from developmental tasks elaborated in G.A.P. Report # 32 and pertain to those young people identified with the official value system. Thus, these indices provide the

clinician with a relative scale to determine how far a young person has progressed.

Emergence from Dependency Status

This is manifested by the ability to relate to parents as co-adults and to work cooperatively with authority figures.

Establishment of Realistic Expectations of People

This is manifested by the ability to form give-and-take relationships.

Control of Ambivalent Feelings

This is manifested by the ability to maintain object relationships despite negative feelings (Farnsworth, 1966; Epstein).

Development of a Personal Value System and Sense of Identity (Laufer, Erikson)

This is the evolutional step following rebellion against the value systems imposed by parents to a point where a personal new code to live by has been developed. The adolescent who persists in life, never having scrutinized and evaluated given rules, but who has accepted noncritically what was given to him is probably still struggling with dependency problems. The adolescent who enters adulthood still preoccupied with the need to challenge authority has not progressed to this phase of autonomous adulthood.

Choice and Pursuit of a Life's Work

This difficult task takes cognizance of the need to find one's interests, preferences and propensities; to successfully compete with others to establish a place for oneself; and to succeed in choosing a life work. The difficulties imposed by a transitional heterogeneous society add to the adolescent's burden.

Ability to Enjoy Sex without Causing Suffering

This would involve removal of inappropriate and anachronistic inhibitions; it would exclude sadomasochistic and exploitative sexual activity; it would engender feelings of love, responsibility and consideration; and it would serve to prolong and enrich a relationship.

Ability to View Life Actively and in Terms of a Series of Problems That Must Inevitably Arise and Be Solved (Grinker)

Evaluation of the Adolescent Mental Status, Including the Clinicians's Intuitive Response

It was noted that young people in the transitional years of adolescence manifest many evidences of disturbed psychology and behavior which are usually short-lived and recede in adulthood. Differentiating them from true, persistent psychopathology or from behavior governed by values of another subculture is taxing and requires clear guidelines and clinical experience.

In attempting to distinguish Masterson's (1968) adolescent turmoil, or what the APA *Diagnostic and Statistical Manual* refers to as the Adjustment Reaction of Adolescence, from true psychopathology, Laufer relies on the following criteria: (1) prior psychiatric history; (2) current level of achievement; (3) success in heterosexual adjustment; (4) the quality and appropriateness of affects, including special note of the degree of sensitivity and proneness to narcissistic injury; (5) the pattern of identifications and whether the idols and companions promote emotional development or regression; and (6) the degree of ego functioning, as illustrated by the ability to distinguish the wish or phantasy from reality and the ability to control impulses when necessary.

Masterson was able to distinguish between relatively sick and relatively healthy adolescents according to their symptomatic picture, scholastic function, social adjustment, and family background. While the more healthy subjects manifested anxiety, depression and obsessive-compulsive traits along with the ill group, these symptoms were sporadic and never became severe fixed patterns. While scholastic function and social adjustment was impaired in the transitionally disturbed group, it was usually minimal, while the sicker patients often showed maximal impairment. Family backgrounds differed, with the transiently disturbed youth coming from broken homes less frequently and having parents and siblings with positive, accepting attitudes.

Machover, viewing adolescent psychopathology psychometrically, concluded that detection of disturbed responses in the projective tests was not of prognostic significance in itself, as adolescents often presented responses that were interpreted as pathological. However, when there was an accompanying decline in intellectual function as well, as measured by intelligence tests, this combination of findings was usually indicative of more serious, persistent mental illness.

Copeland (1964) cites the following criteria as important determiners of the severity of a mental illness: (1) the past psychiatric history; (2) the symptomatic picture; (3) the capacity to function, with comparison between current status and some significant point in the past (inasmuch as academic function is one of the chief barometers of overall function, comparison of the previous year's grades with current ones is often helpful); (4) object relationships in terms of their extensiveness and positive qualities; and (5) the experienced clinician's intuitive or "gut response" to the patient. While this indicator may be no more than a reflection of the clinician's bias and idiosyncrasies, thereby rendering his diagnosis inaccurate, it may have important prognostic significance. The therapist's attitude towards the young patient is often a critical variable in the patient's response to treatment.

RESUME OF KEY FACTORS IN THE PSYCHOLOGICAL EVALUATION OF ADOLESCENTS

Clinical judgment about the mental health or illness of an adolescent is contingent upon direct and indirect factors.

Direct Factors

Symptoms

Sporadic symptoms of anxiety, depression, cyclothymia,

obsessionalism and compulsivity are not in themselves pathognomnic of chronic mental illness. Schizophrenic-like symptoms, such as hallucinations, delusions, or concretistic thinking, are usually correlated with serious future psychopathology. Symptoms that are formed into relatively fixed patterns are also related to future mental illness, while symptoms that are sporadic and loosely organized are usually less serious.

Function

Impaired function in the absence of a demonstrable external stress usually denotes psychopathology. In the face of stress, impairment should be temporary depending upon the severity of the pressure in question. An illustration of this is the incoming college freshman away from home for the first time, who often functions below his academic level for the first semester or two. With the passage of time, however, he is usually able to adapt and once again achieve optimal academic performance.

For the adolescent, impaired function may take the form of academic decline, dropping out of school, frequent job changes, or unemployment.

Object Relations

Prolonged inability to relate to peers, both same-sex and opposite-sex, often suggests psychological illness. Pathological and regressive relationships, involving essentially destructive, perverted or anachronistic behavior is also suggestive of abnormality. Hostile dependency upon family at the expense of peer relationships or total withdrawal from everyone may be indicative of psychological problems.

The Clinician's Intuitive Response

The intuitive response on the part of the experienced and objective clinician is often a valuable indicator of the young patient's condition and prognosis. This response is, in part, a reflection of the clinician's therapeutic expectation and approach, partially a response to his aggregate clinical findings, and in part a response to factors which are probably unconscious, operant both in the patient and in the therapist.

Good feelings about a patient on the part of the seasoned clinician may well indicate a favorable prognosis ultimately, while strong feelings of hopelessness could easily reflect serious mental illness and/or a guarded prognosis.

Indirect Factors

Past Psychological Adjustment

A history of prior psychiatric treatment, major psycho-physiologic illness, use of psychotropic drugs prescribed by the family doctor, "nervous breakdowns," drug abuse, and evidence of prior functional or social impairment would cast a current adolescent psychological problem in a more serious light and incline the clinician to regard the current adolescent turmoil with more gravity.

Family History

A young person experiencing current emotional difficulty and coming from a family that is either broken or demonstrably disturbed is more likely to develop true psychological problems than someone living in a family that appears whole, wholesome, and devoid of apparent major psychopathology.

Psychological Test Results

Abnormal projective test responses in the face of impaired intellectual function is considered more serious prognostically than abnormal projective results with intact intellectual function.

The experienced clinician will take all of the above factors into consideration in deciding how well or how sick his young patient is. Weighing all of the above factors judiciously does not lend itself to easy quantification. However, all patients might be categorized as probably mentally healthy, probably mentally ill, and marginal.

Adequate follow-up with or without treatment will ultimately clarify the status of the "marginal" patient; the adolescent diagnosed as mentally healthy can be reassured and invited to reestablish therapeutic contact if a need arises in the future. Prompt treatment should be instituted for the mentally ill adolescent.

SUMMARY

The concept of the normal adolescent requires much clarification. Meaningful clinical judgments require thorough understanding of adolescent psychology and societal stresses as well as manifestations of adolescent psychopathology.

Seemingly aberrant behavior, rather than reflecting an intrapsychic psychological disturbance, may reflect stress coming from some external source such as the family or the society or the norms of a particular subculture subscribed to by a young person. Seemingly aberrant behavior often is usual and phase-specific, reflecting the stress of the transitional psychophysiological phase of adolescence and waning in adulthood.

The "normal" adolescent, then, is psychologically and behaviorally different from the adult and must be viewed according to adolescent and not adult standards. Persistence of some of the adolescent traits into adult life, however, would constitute psychopathology in some cases, e.g. preoccupation with phantasy life or cyclothymia.

The "normal" adolescent is one

who functions well in his context;

who is capable of personal achievement;

who chooses and keeps friends;

who is oriented more towards adaptation and productivity than towards regression;

who is beginning to relate sexuality to meaningful durable relationships with members of the opposite sex;

who is able to relate to parents less as the dependent minor and more as the cooperative peer;

who frequently manifests symptoms of anxiety and depression sporadically and in a loosely organized way and who might show other neurotic symptoms in the same way;

who evokes positive, optimistic feelings on the part of the seasoned clinician who examines him;

whose psychological test results do not show intellectual impairment in the face of abnormal responses in projective testing.

In cases of doubt, the presence of an intact and psychologically healthy family and the history of health and successful development prior to the adolescent phase suggest a lighter rather than a more serious psychological disturbance. In the final analysis, judgment about an adolescent's normality is a clinical one requiring experience. The above parameters may serve as a guide.

BIBLIOGRAPHY

Aichorn, A.: Wayward Youth. New York, Viking Pr, 1935. American Society for Adolescent Psychiatry, in Newsletter. New York, Apr 1971.

Balser, B.: Psychotherapy of the Adolescent. New York, Int Univs Pr, 1957.

Blos, P.: On Adolescence. New York, Free Pr, 1962.

Caplan, G.: A community mental health program for adolescents. In Caplan, G., and Lebovici, S. (Eds.): Adolescence: Psychosocial Perspectives. New York, Basic, 1969.

Copeland, A.: Determining the severity of mental disorders. Postgraduate Medicine, 6:571-576, 1964.

Eissler, R.: Searchlights on delinquency. In Eissler, R. (Ed.): New Psychoanalytic Studies. New York, Int Univs Pr, 1949.

Escoll, P.: The history of adolescent psychiatry in Philadelphia. Trans Stud Coll Physicians Phila, 35:111-116, 1967-1969.

Farnsworth, D.: Psychiatry Education and the Young Adult. Springfield, Thomas, 1966.

Freud, A.: Adolescence. In Eissler, R. (Ed.): Psychoanalytic Study of the Child. New York, Int Univs Pr, 1958, vol. XIII, pp. 146-151. 1958.

Healy, W., and Bronner, A.: New Light on Delinquency and Its Treatment. New Haven, Institute of Human Relations, 1936.

Johnson, A.: Juvenile delinquency. In Arietti, S. (Ed.): American Handbook of Psychiatry. New York, Basic, 1959, pp. 840-856.

Joint Information Service: The Community Mental Health Center: Analysis of Existing Models. Washington, D.C., 1964.

Josselyn, I.: Adolescents: Everyone's special concern. Int J Psychiatry, 5:465-470, 1968.

Kenniston, K.: Postadolescence (youth) and historical change. In Zubin, J., and Freedman, A. (Ed.): The Psychopathology of Adolescence. New York, Grune, 1970.

Masterson, J.: The old order changeth. Int J Psychiatry, 5:486-491, 1968.

Mora, G.: In Zubin, J., and Freedman, A. (Eds.): The Psychopathology of Adolescence. New York, Grune, 1970, p. 15.

Muus, R.: Theories of Adolescence, 2nd ed. New York, Random, 1968.

Offer, D., and Sabshin, M.: Normality: Theoretical and Clinical Concepts of Mental Health. New York, Basic, 1966.

Piaget, J.: The intellectual development of the adolescent. In Caplan, G., and Lebovici, S. (Eds.): Adolescence: Psychosocial Perspectives. New York, Basic, 1969, pp. 22-27.

Rosen, G.: The revolt of youth: Some historical comparisons. In Zubin, J., and Freedman, A. (Eds.): The Psychopathology of Adolescence. New York, Grune, 1970, pp. 1-14.

Schoenfeld, W.: The adolescent in contemporary American psychiatry. Int J Psychiatry, 5:470-478, 1968.

Schoenfeld, W.: Psychiatry and the adolescent patient: A reply to the critics. Int J Psychiatry, 6:77-79, 1968.

Staples, H.: Modern psychiatry for the adolescent. Int J Psychiatry, 5:492-496, 1968.

Weiss, E.: Emotional memories and acting out. Psychoanal, 11:477, 1942.

What the U.S. will be like in 1980: Meaning of population shifts. U.S. News and World Report, :38-45, Jan., 1971.

Young, H.: Special needs of adolescents. Int J Psychiatry, 5:494-495, 1968.

Zubin, J.: and Freedman, A.: The Psychopathology of Adolescence. New York, Grune, 1970.

CHAPTER III

PSYCHOPATHOLOGY OF ADOLESCENCE

INTRODUCTION

AT this point in time, description and codification of the psychopathological disturbances of adolescence is incomplete. Much clinical work is being done in the field, however, and as more data is accumulated, a wider conceptual frame of reference and an expanded nomenclature will be developed to accomodate this new information.

The Diagnostic and Statistical Manual of the American Psychiatric Association (DSMII, 1968) presents a preliminary adolescent nosology. To date, it is incomplete and relatively unsophisticated conceptually (Wilson, 1971).

While DSMII does recognize the stressfullness of the adolescent phase and the transitional nature of many symptoms and signs, it does not acknowledge the importance of multiple etiology, the family, or subculture and societal influences. DSMII pays insufficient attention to developmental patterns of adolescence, and deviations from these patterns, as forms of psychopathology. Some common psychological and psychosocial syndromes are not included, such as self-mutilation or alienation.

Behavioral disturbances of childhood and adolescence are listed as one category. Many of these problems are, however, phase specific and should not be listed together. For example, the group delinquent reaction is usually a post-pubertal phenomenon not seen much in children; hyperkinesis, on the other hand, is usually found in children and not found in that form in adolescents.

Subsequent revisions of the Diagnostic and Statistical Manual might well include a separate section on adolescent psychopathology.

BASIC CONCEPTS

1. The adolescent viewed as mentally ill may be perceived as such for a variety of reasons: he may be manifesting symptoms of deep-seated psychological problems; he may be essentially reacting to a period of developmental stress; he may be identifying with the values of a particular subculture; he may be reacting to family or societal stress; he may be adjudged mentally sick by virtue of the bias of the observer; he may be seen as mentally ill for any combination of the above factors.

2. Social and genetic factors as well as psychological factors must be considered as etiological forces in many cases; and knowledge of family dynamics, peer group values, societal pressures, and biogenetic factors are essential.

3. From a psychological standpoint, psychopathology may arise by virtue of deprivation, deficiency and default or via conflict, with resulting anxiety and neurosis. (Chodoff, 1972.)

4. Clinical and developmental concepts of what is normative and what is pathological must be understood. The mentally ill adolescent is generally characterized by maladaptive or bizarre behavior, affect, thinking, attitudes and/or function.

5. Psychopathological manifestations in adolescence are often more labile than adult conditions and more easily revised. Thus, the term "disturbances" should be employed to denote the lability and prognostic uncertainty of these conditions.

6. Severity of symptoms is not necessarily related to the seriousness of the disturbances or their prognosis.

7. Early recognition and vigorous treatment of all of the etiological roots to an adolescent disturbance have an important effect upon prognosis. The amount of ego strength, positive accomplishments, and family support available are also important.

8. Current nosology is generally inadequate in that it is descriptively incomplete and conceptually unsophisticated. A complete nosology should include descriptive, psychodynamic, familial, cultural and biological etiological factors and indicate their relative importance.

9. The term "schizophrenoid disturbance" should be employed to differentiate it from the term "schizophrenia" which would

incorrectly create the impression of homogeneity, fixity and guarded prognosis.

10. The "Group Delinquent Reaction of Adolescence," cited in DSMII, could be divided into two categories:

a) *Violent Group Delinquent Disturbance,* considered destructive behavior, and

b) *Minor Group Delinquent Disturbance,* a condition much more ubiquitous and less pathologic.

The following system has been devised as an initial attempt towards the development of an adolescent nosology.

CLASSIFICATION

   I. Developmental Disturbances
      A. Fixation – Regression Disturbances
      B. Identity Disturbances
         1. Basic Identity Disturbance
         2. Gender Identity Disturbance
            Homosexuality
  II. Adjustment Reaction of Adolescence
 III. Neurotoid Disturbances
 IV. Affective Disturbances
      A. Normative Cyclothymia
      B. Depressive Disturbances
         1. Depressiveness
         2. Depressive Equivalents
         3. Depressive Suicidal Behavior
      C. Anxiety
      D. Guilt
      E. Other
   V. Behavior Disturbances
      A. Flight
         1. Runaway
         2. Withdrawal
      B. Destructive Behavior Disturbances
         1. Unsocialized Aggressive Disturbance
         2. Violent Group Delinquent Disturbance
         3. Self-mutilation

      4. Suicidal Behavior (Nondepressive)
      5. Psychogenic Accidents
      6. Homicidal Behavior
   C. Heterosexual Behavior Disturbances
      1. Withdrawal/Asceticism
      2. Promiscuity/Prostitution
      3. Psychopathological Pregnancy
      4. Male Sexual Dysfunction
  VI. Pharmacopathia
  VII. Schizophrenoid Disturbance
VIII. Psychosocial Disturbances
   A. Family-Unit Disturbance
   B. Alienation Disturbance
   C. Minor Group Delinquent Disturbance
  IX. Psychophysiological Disturbances
   A. Anorexia Nervosa
   B. Obesity
   C. Headache
   D. Ulcerative Colitis – Regional Enteritis
   E. Asthma
   F. Enuresis

Developmental Disturbances

Description

These are psychological problems of adolescence directly related to unresolved problems of childhood and manifested by behavior and symptoms which are more characteristic of childhood than of youth.

Two kinds of problems will be described: Fixation-Regression Disturbances or "childishness" and Identity Disturbances or problems of "who am I – what am I?"

Fixation-Regression Disturbances

Fixations

These are defined as behavior patterns or symptom complexes that are anachronistic and have persisted from an earlier period in childhood where they were more appropriate or adaptive. For instance, bed-wetting or enuresis noted in the young child is considered fixational if it persists past five years of age (Murphy and Chapman, 1970). Other manifestations of fixation may be masochism or the quest for pain, defeat or humiliation (Borawitz, 1971); narcissism or self-centeredness (Rose, 1971; Garmezy, 1970); homosexuality (Giovacchini, 1971); and passive-dependency (Kahn, 1971).

Regressions

These are explained as patterns of behavior or symptom complexes that reappear from an earlier phase of development after a dormant period. Regressions may be adaptive, such as temporary withdrawal, as a means of coping with strong and dangerous impulses (Esson, 1971). They may be maladaptive, as with thumbsucking. Other forms of regression are hypersensitivity, slovenliness or destructiveness (Sklansky, 1969); secondary enuresis (DeLuca, 1968); obsessionalism or compulsivity and anorexia nervosa in boys (Jochmus, 1967).

Etiologically, regressions are believed to be precipitated by some form of stress occurring in adolescence superimposed upon earlier unresolved problems of development.

Fixations persisting in adolescence are also believed to reflect early developmental disturbances such as deprivations and/or psychological trauma occurring in the mother-child relationship (Maney; Chodoff, 1972). Stresses in the family and the surrounding culture also contribute.

Prognostically, self-depreciating traits may be more easy to treat than traits of self-indulgence, assaultiveness, withdrawal or bizarreness (Garmezy, 1970).

Sklansky (1969) distinguishes the regression of adolescence from the more serious preschizophrenic disorders by its temporary nature, its unacceptability to the adolescent, and the integrity and continued function of the rest of his personality in the face of regression.

Treatment of regressive and fixational disturbances depends upon how severe and disruptive they are. As already indicated, fixations that do not interfere with the general course of psychological development do not require treatment. Regressions that serve as temporary coping mechanisms without disrupting emotional growth may be strengthened or left alone.

On the other hand, regressions and fixations that are maladaptive or destructive must be dealt with. Psychotherapy is helpful; and selection of a particular approach, whether individual, group or family therapy, must be determined on an individual basis.

Identity Disturbances

Description

Identity is a sense of self predicated upon the achievement of stable personal values and integrated actions. A sense of identity is consistent with the conviction that life makes sense (Milstein, 1971).

Problems of adolescent identity focus upon such questions as "who am I?", "what am I?", "what should I do?", and "what should I become?"

A rudimentary self-awareness in the infant arises from the perception of his bodily functions and limits which eventually produces a body image (Hoffer, 1949). A conducive mother-infant relationship further aids the child in differentiating himself from her and the rest of the world and establishing himself as a unique entity (Mahler, 1963). Progress in identity formation made during childhood is often slowed by the stresses of adolescence. Fundamental changes in the young person's biology and psychology coupled with a number of new social pressures often produce disturbances in his sense of identity.

Two kinds of identity disturbances will be described: Basic Identity Disturbance and Gender Identity Disturbance.

Basic Identity Disturbance

Description. This is a period of acute anxiety and depression borne of an urgent sense of self-doubt and the uncertainty about "who am I — what am I?" (Erikson, 1959). Symptomatically, there is a complaint of feelings of diffuseness and uncertainty. Behavior, thinking and values may be highly erratic and inconsistent as well.

Etiologically, the psycho-biosociological stresses of adolescence coupled with unresolved problems of childhood produce this crisis of "who am I — what am I?"

Basic identity crises may be differentiated from schizophrenoid psychosis by (1) the continued capacity to relate to others; (2) the absence of bizarreness; (3) the temporary nature of the identity crisis; (4) the maintenance of an inner nucleus of personality intactness and a sense of reality, despite the superficial identity diffusion (Blaine, 1971; Sklansky, 1969).

Treatment consists of psychotherapy which will support existing areas of personality intactness, reduce the level of anxiety, and provide a psychological anchor at a time of uncertainty and crisis.

Gender Identity Disturbance

Description. A confusion about or conflict with one's biological gender. One's sense of masculinity of femininity constitutes an important part of the individual's total identity (Shainess, 1972). Basic notions regarding one's sexual identity are derived from biological constitutional factors as well as family upbringing (Garmazy, 1970; Goldberg, 1972), and this sense of masculinity or femininity is a partly unconscious phenomenon.

Psychobiological aspects of Male and Female Identity. A. Freud, Deutsch and others have written about particular psychologies associated with men and women. While Freud characterized women as passive and masochistic and men as aggressive, Shainess (1972), Erickson (1968) and others modify this view and characterize that which is female as receptive and enveloping and that which is masculine as penetrating.

To better understand differences in the perspectives and psychologies of men and women, it is important to review their psychobiological developments. From a statistical standpoint, there is a higher rate of conception, intrauterine mortality, and birth for males; the reasons are imperfectly understood. Yet male intrauterine mortality is 12 percent higher than the female and there are 106 males born for every 100 human females (Adam and Eve, 1972).

Embryological development is different chronologically for each gender with testicular formation occurring in the male around the sixth week and with ovary formation occurring around the twelfth week. Palate closure and eye and teeth formation occur sooner in the male as well (Katz, 1972). There is also evidence to believe that fetal androgens stimulate a peculiarly masculine organization of brain tissue, eventually producing a peculiarly masculine behavior (Jost, 1953; Money 1970).

In the newborn, males and females are morphologically different, with boys being huskier and having larger frames and limbs. Newborn males raise their heads higher than females. Baby girls, on the other hand, show a greater light-sensitivity and interest in touching. In addition they show a greater resistance to infections, probably on the basis of their bearing an extra "X" chromosome, the site of immunoglobulin synthesis (Gadpaille, 1973).

In childhood, physical development is gender-specific with the female growth spurt occurring at around nine-and-one-half years of age and that of the male at eleven-and-one-half years (Sklansky, 1969). There is also evidence that females display better visual motor coordination than males (Gilbert, 1969).

In the adolescent phase, male behavior is more kinetic and exhibitionistic while the female focuses upon tenderness, falling in love, and being loved (Sklansky, 1969).

Sexually, the male is most active between the ages of sixteen and twenty (Kinsey, et al., 1948) while the female reaches her peak at least a decade later (Athanasiou, 1973).

In attempting to delineate an exclusively female psychology, Shainess (1972) points to exclusively feminine life experiences that influence her thinking: menarche, breast development, defloration, delivery and menopause. The act of sexual intercourse represents very different experiences for the male and the female. Many authors have pointed out the dramatic impact that the menstrual flow has upon the psychology of the female (Deutsch,

Glass, et al., 1971; Dalton, 1964). The male experience is unique as well, with an orgastic function that is solitary rather than multiple and a capacity for erection and copulation that is reliant upon conducive psychological conditions to a large degree (Masters and Johnson, 1966). No such preconditions can absolutely control female copulation.

On the basis of unique psychobiological differences in development, morphology, and function, a gender-specific perspective and identity crystalizes and constitutes a significant part of one's total identity.

While social values importantly influence the roles and functions of men and women, psychobiological forces render the masculine and feminine genders unique and distinct.

Biological Disorders Related to Disturbances of Gender Identity. Gender-identity disturbances may be caused by biological problems, although psychological factors appear to be of greater importance (Money, 1970). Among these biological factors are chromosomal aberrations, hormonal imbalance, and gonadal abnormalities, as well as abnormalities of the external genitalia.

The following syndromes are illustrative:

1. *Testicular Feminizing Syndrome.* This condition is characterized by the presence of external female genitals and internal testicles. The biological problem is that of androgen failure in the presence of a normal chromosomal pattern. Individuals with testicular feminizing syndrome are usually feminine psychobiologically and seek male sexual partners.

2. *Klinefelter's Syndrome.* In this condition there are atrophic testes and small male genitalia present in young males who look considerably younger than their chronological age. They may manifest gynecomastia, appear psychotic, or come to the attention of a physician because of sterility. This condition is believed attributable to a chromosomal aberration: XXY. They are psychologically masculine and usually seek female sex partners.

3. *Turner's Syndrome (Ovarian Dysgenesis).* Girls with Turner's syndrome are usually short and fail to undergo pubertal changes. This condition occurs with a statistical frequency of 1/2000 to 1/3000 and is attributable to the absence of an X chromosome.

Biologically and psychologically, such individuals are usually female.

Another condition may be noted in individuals with an XXX chromosomal pattern who are believed to have a variable psychosexual identity and sexual activity pattern (Money, 1970).

Psychological and Sociological Factors Related to Disturbances of Gender Identity. While biological problems may produce conflict and confusion about one's sense of masculinity or femininity, most individuals with disturbances of gender identity have no demonstrable organic problem (Katz, 1972).

Both Baker and Stoller (1968) point out the importance of psychological as well as biological factors and Money (1970) stresses the importance of early childhood experiences.

Katz (1972) finds the following factors important in the development of gender identity: (1) the nature of the mother-infant dyad during the first one-and-one-half years; (2) the toilet training experience; (3) the child's name; (4) the child's dress; (5) parental attitudes regarding aggressivity; (6) parental seductiveness; (7) roles assigned to the child; (8) the role of the same-sex parent in fostering identification.

Homosexuality and Gender Identity Disturbance. Homosexuality will be defined as the obligatory quest for sexual interaction with someone of the same gender. It may be borne of a deep-seated gender identity disturbance in which homosexual behavior is a defense against a more painful and difficult-to-handle heterosexuality (Sklansky, 1969).

Homosexual behavior may reflect the values of a particular subculture, e.g. a prison population. It may reflect experimentation in sex amongst neophytes, and it may be a manifestation of expediency, as noted in Russell's study of boy prostitutes.

Thus, homosexual behavior among adolescents does not necessarily indicate a serious psychological problem (Goldberg, 1972). However, adequate evaluation is necessary to assure prompt treatment if necessary. In those adolescents whose homosexuality reflects a true gender identity disturbance, maternal seductiveness and over-protectiveness seem to play an important etiological role, both for boys (Giovacchini, 1971) and girls (Borawitz, 1971).

124547

Manifestations of Gender Identity Disturbances. A disturbance in one's sense of masculinity or femininity may manifest itself in a variety of ways. The following symptoms and behavioral patterns are associated with gender identity disturbance but are not at all pathognomonic. It is important to weigh all factors before arriving at such a diagnosis, for misdiagnosis in this area of exquisite sensitivity to the adolescent may produce needless harm and suffering. Thus, it is essential for the clinician to go beyond the presenting symptoms listed below before arriving at a diagnosis of gender identity disturbance:

1. Effeminacy in the male and "tom-boyism" in the female
2. Transvestitism (Newman, 1970)
3. Homosexual behavior (Giovacchini, 1971)
4. Female promiscuity, assaultiveness and thievery (Milstein, 1971; Felsenberg).
5. Self-mutilation (Rosenthal, et al., 1972)
6. Violence
7. Drug addiction (Chwast, 1971)
8. Dysmenorrhea (Copeland)
9. Anorexia Nervosa (Bruch)

Thus the presence of any of the symptoms or syndromes requires a thorough psychiatric evaluation of their significance. They must not be ignored.

Differential Diagnosis. 1. *Superficial opposite-sex identification.* This is illustrated by the boy who shows superficial effeminate behavior by virtue of identification with a significant female in his life and on a deeper level has a true masculine identity and non-conflicted heterosexual strivings.

2. *Maternal deprivation.* Russell (1971) describes transitional homosexual behavior in maternally-deprived boys in response to exploitative homosexual men. This behavior is temporary, however, and not indicative of a true disturbance of gender identity.

3. *Social mores.* Behavior that may be considered indicative of gender identity conflict may simply reflect adolescent compliance with contemporary peer-group values. The switch from short hair to long in the male and the predilection for pants rather than skirts in the female are illustrative of such compliance.

Homosexual behavior in a juvenile correctional facility may also reflect institutional mores rather than true disturbances of gender identity.

4. *Regression.* Sklansky (1969) describes temporary regression away from threatening heterosexual impulses and the adoption of transitional homosexual behavior in the adolescent. Mutual exploring and masturbation have been noted in early adolescence and usually abate in later adolescence.

Therapeutic Considerations. One of the initial tasks of psychotherapy is to help define for the adolescent this conflict associated with masculinity or femininity. Shame and fear often impede such definition, requiring much tact and patience on the part of the therapist.

A relationship that is conducive to identifying with the desired qualities of the same-sex therapist is very important. If gender definition by example with the same-sex therapist is effective, gender definition by contrast and encouragement by a therapist of the opposite sex can be valuable as well. Thus same-sex and opposite-sex therapists can be effective.

In less profound disturbances of gender identity, supportive identifications alone, without profound intrapsychic probing, are sufficient. Only the most experienced therapists should deal with the deeper psychodynamics of gender identity disturbances in the adolescent. Family therapy and/or removal from a noxious environment may also be indicated.

Prognosis. Prognosis is greatly influenced by timing. The earlier the therapeutic intervention, the better the result. Newman (1970) notes that for the transexual, however, persistence of the wish to be accepted as a member of the opposite sex past childhood renders the therapeutic task more difficult.

Adjustment Reaction of Adolescence

The *Diagnostic and Statistical Manual* of the American Psychiatric Association (DSM II, 1968) describes the "Adjustment Reaction of Adolescence" as a transitional situational disorder characterized by irritability, depression, temper outbursts, brooding, and discouragement associated with school failure. It may reach psychotic proportions in the face of sufficient stress and recede where the stress diminishes. Blaine (1971) notes that all kinds of symptoms may be noted in this condition; he includes hypomania, drug misuse, stealing, etc.

If the symptoms persist and disrupt the overall personality development and function, however, another diagnosis should be considered.

Neurotoid Disturbances

Neurotoid disturbances of the adolescent are descriptively the same as the neuroses of the adult, as described in DSM II. While they connote the same symptoms and syndromes, they do not necessarily reflect the same fixity, severity or prognosis. On the contrary, early and appropriate therapeutic intervention often leads to rapid improvement. Thus "neurotoid disturbance" is used in place of neurosis to denote adolescent psychopathology that is more labile than that of the adult.

The neurotoid disturbances include hysterical neurosis, phobic neurosis, obsessive compulsive neurosis, depressive neurosis, neurasthenic neurosis, depersonalization neurosis, and hypochondriacal neurosis. Obsessionalism or compulsivity may be considered a regression-fixation disturbance when regression or fixation can be demonstrated. Anxiety and depression may be considered affective disturbances when they are more a transitory reaction to a period of developmental stress and less a reflection of underlying organized psychopathology. Anxiety, depression, obsessionalism and compulsivity may be considered simply manifestations of adolescent stress. (see Ch. II)

Affective Disturbances

Description

Affective disturbances of adolescence are common and are manifestations of developmental stress. Common affective disturbances of young people are cyclothymia, depression, anxiety, anger and guilt (Masterson, 1970). No doubt others exist and will be described subsequently.

Cyclothymia and Normal Adolescence

Mood swings alternating between "feeling low" and exuberance are frequent occurrences that can be triggered by apparently minor victories and defeats in the life of the young person. Moods may swing sharply and unpredictably during the course of a day or week. They are short-lived and not disruptive of personality development or function.

"Normal" cyclothymia may be differentiated from manic depression by the absence of a bipolar depressive history in the family, the absence of personality disruptions, and the patient's capacity to perceive the mood swings as atypical and alien. In addition, manic-depressives often show a pattern of over-compliance to authority figures and preoccupation with ideas of guilt and impending loss (Arietti, 1959).

Depressive Disturbances

Depressiveness

Frank adolescent depressiveness is similar to that of the adult form with sadness of mood; a negative, derogatory sense of self; convictions of helplessness and hopelessness; and ideas of rejection. In addition, there may be altered body functions such as seen in anorexia nervosa as well as the loss of libido (Blaine, 1971; Masterson, 1970). Academic function is often impaired and may lead to failure and school withdrawal (Hollan, 1970; Whitney, 1971).

The following poem was written by a thirteen-year-old girl hospitalized after having run away from a correctional institution where she had been placed by rejecting parents. The tone of hopelessness and helplessness is pervasive. Some glimmer of hope emerges in the end, however.

Life for Me is Dead and Gone

Life for me is dead and gone
And I don't know where I could have gone wrong.
I don't have a mother
(and I don't think I'm allowed to have another).
I don't have a father
(I guess they're too much bother).

I don't have sisters or brothers
(I guess we don't need each other).
I'm just thirteen and have a long way to go,
And I know I have to grow.
I have to push forth like a seed in the sun,
Not knowing the meaning of fun.
I have to grow big, smart and tall,
And I've got to be better than the rest of them all.
I've got to grow mean and have lots of wits,
Not grow like a baby who has lots of fits.
But life for me is dead and gone.
And I don't know where I could have gone wrong.

Depressive Equivalents

Depressive equivalents are atypical, masked forms of frank depression appearing commonly in adolescence and frequently taking a behavioral or psychophysiological form.

Masterson (1970) cites destructive acting out as an equivalent of depression and Finch (1972) and Toolan (1969) include restlessness and overeating. Ling et al. (1970) note the importance of headache, withdrawal, and the presence of persecutory ideas; and Frederick (1972) cites fatigue in this connection. Inexplicable outbursts of aggression and "meanness" may also reflect an inner depressiveness: academic dysfunction has been noted, and a pattern of accidents may also be considered in this light.

Case. Cindy was a fifteen-year-old girl hospitalized for her uncontrollable outbursts of anger. Initially, she presented as a hostile and aggressive adolescent who was constantly on the attack. With time, her positive adjustment to the inpatient unit made her hostility increasingly inappropriate and unacceptable to her. Upon the subsidance of her aggressivity she became frankly depressive. Her essential defense against depression as well as her depressive equivalent was gone, revealing the underlying affective pathology.

Depressive Suicidal Behavior

Suicidal behavior is common in adolescence — the fifth leading cause of death in the 15 to 19 year age group (Kraus, 1972). While comparable behavior in the adult is considered intimately related to depression, this is not necessarily so in the adolescent population.

Balser, Masterson and Blaine (1959) consider suicidal behavior at this phase closely associated with schizophrenia; Finch (1972) links it to character disorders; and Beal (1969) views suicide as a psychosocial phenomenon with multiple etiological roots. Identification with someone who is suicidal also plays an important role (Rostov, 1970). Thus suicidal behavior in young people is complex and probably not as closely associated with depression as in the adult. Suicidal behavior will be further discussed under "Destructive Behavior Disturbance."

Anxiety Disturbance

Anxiety is a psychophysiologic response (comparable to that of fear) to a non-external, intra-psychic stress. It is characterized by the subjective feeling of uneasiness, fear, dread, or a sense of impending danger. It produces a readiness to flee or fight in the individual along with a variety of physiological manifestations affecting a number of organ systems:

1. Cardiovascular, e.g. tachycardia
2. Pulmonary, e.g. hyperventilation
3. Gastrointestinal, e.g. nausea, vomiting and fecal incontinence
4. Genito-urinary, e.g. urinary incontinence
5. Tegumentary, e.g. sweating
6. Gynecological, e.g. amenorrhea
7. Musculoskeletal, e.g. muscle spasm

Anxiety is believed to be the basis for the development of adult neurosis (DSM II, 1968).

The anxiety disturbance of adolescence is presently subsumed under "Neurosis" and "Over-anxious Reaction of Childhood and Adolescence" in DSM II. Under this latter category are included the symptoms of insomnia and nightmares as well as the personality traits of inhibition, compliance and self-consciousness.

Anxiety disturbance must be differentiated from the characteristic and ever-present anxiety that is so conspicuous in adolescence. In general, when anxiety is sufficient to impair personality function, object relations, and psychological development, it is considered an anxiety disturbance.

Anxiety in the presence of neurotic symptoms will be considered part of that neurotoid disturbance of adolescence.

Guilt Disturbance

This is a psychological condition characterized by a crisis of conscience and the pervading feeling of having done something wrong along with the accompanying conviction of being hated as a consequence. There is often denial of instinctual impulses, especially sexual, and a general curtailment of activities and heterosexual relationships although same-sex companionships may be maintained.

Case. Jane was an eighteen-year-old high school graduate brought to the psychiatrist by her mother because of nervousness, loss of appetite and insomnia. She presented the initial appearance of a girl in great discomfort and pain and spoke almost inaudibly about her guilt and shame. She felt mortified and apparently could find no place to hide.

Her guilt was compounded by her avoidance of church, as she could not face confessing the sins that were torturing her so. In therapy, she would continually ask the therapist if he hated her. After several months of treatment, she became aware of the close association between her feelings of sinfulness and self-hatred on the one hand, and her erotic feelings and frankly sexual dreams. Control of these impulses was not mediated by reason and strength of personality but rather by a conscience that was harsh and sadistic and which made her feel dirty and despicable. Jane's solution to the demands of her drives and the recriminations of conscience was to embark on a life of spartan asceticism. She withdrew from all pleasures including food, friends and even school which meant so much to her. During the course of therapy Jane gradually resumed her psychological growth and moved stepwise back into the mainstream of life when she was able to accept the universality of her feelings and the inevitability of her adulthood.

Intense guilt is not uncommon in adolescence and may appear as such or in an equivalent form such as asceticism or by acting out with the quest for punishment.

Guilt disturbances may be differentiated from a schizoid personality disorder and simple schizophrenia by the absence of bizarreness and the intactness of the rest of the personality.

Jane presented features of both disorders. Her cessation of academic function and impoverishment of social relationships, which became progressive, suggested a schizophrenoid process. Her withdrawal, shyness, daydreaming and sensitivity pointed towards a schizoid disorder or withdrawal disturbance of adolescence. However, psychopathology in the adolescent phase is frequently more labile than that of its adult counterpart, frequently rendering a better though more unpredictable prognosis. Vigorous therapeutic intervention may dramatically reverse a pattern of regression and total personality breakdown.

Jane's guilt disturbance became an isolated phenomenon of diminishing importance.

Behavior Disturbances

Description

These are nonadaptive and/or destructive patterns of behavior in response to the internal and external stresses of the adolescent phase. The *Diagnostic and Statistical Manual* includes overactivity, inattentiveness, shyness, feelings of rejection, over-aggressiveness, timidity and delinquency in this category. Behavior disturbances will be classified here in terms of the adolescent's pathologic behavior response to disturbing sexual and aggressive impulses which he has difficulty in mediating:
  A. Flight Disturbance
  B. Destructive Behavior Disturbance
  C. Heterosexual Behavior Disturbance
In group A, stress is handled by avoidance. In the second group, aggressive impulses take on a destructive rather than adaptive form. In group C, problems involving heterosexual behavior predominate. While it is quite true that homosexual behavior might have been considered a behavior disturbance in response to instinctual stresses, it was decided to include it under developmental disturbances in order to treat it more fully.

Flight Disturbance

Runaway Reaction

Description. Flight from one's domicile by a minor without knowledge or permission of parents or parental surrogates. Running away is usually in response to an internal, family or subcultural stress and requires careful evaluation of each case. Flight may be a manifestation of psychopathology or a sign of health and strength.

Legal Considerations. According to Herzberg (1972), more than one-half million legal minors run away each year. Upon parental petition to the court, such an act may be punished and a minor remanded to a correctional facility or psychiatric institution. When the runaway adolescent establishes himself independently, the court may regard him as an emancipated minor and not obliged to be returned to the parental domicile or correctional or psychiatric facility. Apparently there is no universal agreement regarding qualification for emancipated minor status. Failure to evaluate individual, family, and social factors adequately may needlessly stigmatize an adolescent as "incorrigible" in his quest to escape from a destructive home or neighborhood environment.

Contemporary Societal Trends. The concept of flight as a societally-approved, temporary respite from external stress seems to be gaining wider acceptance. More and more colleges and universities are allowing students to take official leaves of absence without prejudice in the face of personal need, and this form of approved temporary leave is occurring even at the high school level.

Troubled youth in Samoa enjoyed the option of withdrawal from the immediate family to the domicile of another family member in times of conflict (Mead). Here in the United States, communes have developed which provide refuge for youth under stress, and shelters such as Huckleberry House in San Francisco have sprung up to care for runaways. At this time, legislation has been introduced to provide federal support to local governments to aid these youth. Thus, the runaway is regarded more as someone requiring assistance rather than someone who is incorrigible and needing punishment.

Underlying factors. While the causes of running away are numerous, the following factors are considered important.

1. Feelings of rejection
2. The presence of an unhealthy or threatening situation
3. The flight to a situation believed to be more rewarding (Jenkins, 1971).

DSM II associates stealing, timidity, friendlessness and submissiveness with the runaway. But there are young people with more positive motivation who run away. The following case vignettes are illustrative:

Case 1. Bobby is an eighteen-year-old who fled from a broken and devitalized home to the security and recognition of a gang peer group. His runaway pattern was that of school truancy and periodic absenses from home for two- and three-day periods.

Case 2. Cathy is a fourteen-year-old whose father questioned her legitimacy, rejected her, and punished her arbitrarily. He actively sought institutionalization for her. In response, she stole and ran away.

Case 3. Ann is a thirteen-year-old whose flight took the form of periodic incursions into the "hippy" culture where she was offered shelter and a good time and where she would remain for two and three days. During that time, she would be promiscuous. Her flights and returns to the family fold paralleled the behavior of her father who had left the family several years before to have an affair and who re-entered the family after a period of time.

Treatment of the runaway must include evaluation of the family as well as the adolescent. When these psychotherapeutic overtures are unsuccessful, placement of the young person in a healthier domicile should be explored by all concerned. The mental health field is beginning to become aware of this very important problem of the runaway.

Withdrawal Disturbance

Description. This is a flight reaction characterized by its transient nature, the preference for solitude, shyness and sensitivity in the presence of others, and the avoidance of close personal friendships (DSMII, 1968). The function of the withdrawal is considered defensive in nature, providing the adolescent the opportunity to take stock of himself and "regroup" or reorganize his psychological defenses before going forth to test his new self in the challenging world of adult drives (Sklansky, 1969; Erikson, 1959). The period required for withdrawal varies with the individual and may last for minutes or months.

The withdrawal disturbance is differentiated from schizophrenia by the preservation of ego function and affect in the face of withdrawal. In addition, there is preservation of interest in the outside world during the period of retreat. Differentiation from a schizoid disorder is difficult, but the former is a more transitory disturbance.

From a therapeutic standpoint, it is essential to ascertain the psychodynamic factors involved. If the withdrawal is simply a regressive defense against adolescent stress, the relationship with a supportive therapist is important as it provides the link with the outside world. The therapist can also interpret the adolescent's drives in a less threatening way as well as help smooth out problems of reality. The therapist's role in adolescent withdrawal, then, is essentially supportive.

Destructive Behavior Disturbance

Description

This is a group of behavior patterns and syndromes characterized by overt or covert destructive behavior either to the self or to others.

Unsocialized Aggressive Disturbance

Description. This condition is characterized by challenging, aggressive, and sometimes assaultive behavior both towards peers and adults. In addition, there may be impulsiveness, temper tantrums, lying, stealing and biting (Wilschke, 1968). Such behavior is usually solitary rather than occurring in groups. Etiologically, lack of parental acceptance and discipline are considered important. This condition is to be differentiated from the Violent Group Delinquent Disturbance by its individual, unsocialized, hostile nature.

A therapeutic milieu that fairly sets limits, promotes reflective thinking rather than impulsive behavior, and fosters positive identifications can be effective.

Violent Group Delinquent Disturbance

Description. A pattern of adolescent peer-group behavior in which violence plays an important and often semi-ritualized role. This violence is often directed against members of rival gangs, although no one is immune. Other aspects of this behavior pattern include the establishment of an elaborate peer-group hierarchy and the demarcation of a territory of "turf" to be defended from the incursions of rival gangs.

The etiological roots (Gutierrez, 1971; Jenkins, 1971) of violent gang behavior are multiple and include psychological, familial and cultural factors. Individual psychopathology among members of violent gangs is not uncommon and includes psychosis and depression as well as problems of passive dependence. In addition there may be organic brain syndrome, a history of encephalitis, and electro-encephalographic changes noted (Beshai, 1971).

The adolescent quest for separation from parental yoke, autonomy and recognition is important as the violent gang bestows just such rewards to its adherents. In the family background there is often parental absence, neglect, and a history of gang membership on the part of one or both parents. The subculture is often devitalized and ghetto-like, walled off from the mainstream of the society, and with a high degree of acceptance of violence as a way of life (Copeland, in press).

While the problem of violent street gangs is complex and does not lend itself to easy solutions, effective approaches lie in the use of gang members with whom the youngster can identify and who, in turn, will divert the gang members into more constructive channels (Reid, personal communication). Development of training and activities programs is helpful; special therapeutic communities and camps have proven effective (Thrasher and Short, 1962; Kelly, 1971).

The Violent Group Delinquent Disturbance is to be differentiated from the more benign "Minor Group Delinquent Disturbances" by the presence of violence and territoriality.

Self-Mutilation

Description. This is composed of diverse patterns of self-inflicted injury associated with different nosological categories and not necessarily suicidal in intent (Mannino and Delgado, 1969).

Self-mutilation may reflect the mores of a subculture which institutionalizes such destructiveness as a means of controlling anxiety. Such behavior has been found among young Peruvian prisoners (Cooper, 1971).

Self-mutilation is noted in schizophrenics with head-banging, a frequent premonitory sign. When associated with problems of gender identity and accompanied by erotization of the act, the prognosis is more guarded (Green, 1967; Mannino and Delgado, 1969).

Several forms of self-mutilation are noteworthy.

1. Trichotillomania, the compulsive drive to pull out hair. It occurs both in males and females who may or may not be psychotic. There is usually no pain associated with the act. The family background frequently reveals an intensely disturbed and close mother-patient dyad (Sanderson and Hall-Smith, 1970).

2. Eye enucleation usually occurs in older people where guilt and depression are primary. It is occasionally noted in adolescents accompanied by psychosis or organic brain damage (Davidson, 1962).

3. Tongue biting and mutilation is seen in adolescent females with diagnoses of psychosis, hysteria or subnormality (Slawson and Davidson, 1965).

4. Autocastration occurs in young males with problems of gender identity, an intense compliant relationship with mother, and the presence of much guilt, shame and anxiety. The act of autocastration is believed to relieve these intensely unpleasant affects (Wong and Blacker).

5. Skin Slicing is perhaps one of the most common forms of self-mutilation among contemporary adolescents. The adolescent

is usually an attractive female. The site of injury is usually the wrist or forearm, although slashes have been observed on the hand, thigh and ankle as well. Skin slicers fall under a variety of diagnoses including schizophrenia, personality disorder, "borderline state" and hysteria. (Nelson, 1971; Grunebaum and Klerman, 1967; Mannino and Delgado, 1969). Background features include early maternal deprivation (Graff and Mallin, 1967; Rosenthal et al., 1972), parental seduction and incestuous behavior in the family (Grunebaum and Klerman, 1967).

The actual slash is often in response to a sense of loss of an important person or an attempt to manipulate that person. The absence of pain during the slash is often noted and associated with what is believed to be an hysterical anesthesia. The slash brings a sense of relief from internal stresses and personality integration afterwards (Rosenthal et al., 1972).

Therapeutic goals should include the development of better impulse control and acquisition of social skills to combat a common sense of emptiness. The therapeutic approach should include closeness, but never to the point of seductiveness or erotic stimulation. Therapists should be on the alert for attempts to polarize significant authority figures into opposing factions, and constant communication on the part of all concerned is essential. A stormy hospital course fraught with further slashing attempts, infractions of hospital rules, and flight from the hospital often occurs. In successful treatment, impulsive behavior is converted to reflective thought which becomes the basis for therapeutic interaction and psychological growth. Prognosis is guarded when the slash becomes eroticized or reflects guilt in a frankly schizophrenic patient. While many such adolescents improve during the course of hospitalization on an open unit, some may require a more structured setting (Nelson, 1971; Grunebaum and Klerman, 1967).

Inasmuch as skin slicing has several psychodynamic roots, one need not assume suicidal intent until there is sufficient evidence. In order to determine the intent of the patient, close observation, probably in a hospital setting, is indicated.

Suicidal Behavior

Description. Suicidal behavior is defined as overt or covert self-destructive actions that may produce death or injury. It is multietiological and occurs in a variety of socio- and psychopathological conditions.

Incidence. Suicidal behavior among youth seems to be increasing. The incidence of self-inflicted death in the fifteen- to nineteen-year age group rose from 3.6/100,000 in 1960 to 4.7/100,000 in 1967 (Finch and Poznansky, 1971). For each suicidal death, there are fifteen unsuccessful attempts in the overall population (Kraus, 1972), but more than thirty-three attempts in the age group of twenty years and younger (Caplan and Lebovici, 1969).

Males succeed in killing themselves more frequently than females (Otto, 1967); collegians kill themselves at about four times the rate of noncollegians, and this rate is correlated directly with the level of parental education (Blaine, 1971). From a racial standpoint, suicide is more frequent among white youth, although the rate is increasing both among black and white youth populations (Caplan and Lebovici, 1969).

Forms of Suicidal Behavior. Self-destructive behavior may be conscious and willful or may be more covert and take a variety of indirect forms such as pseudo-accidents or drug overdosage (Toolan, 1969). Heavy drug users and suicide attempters have been found to be preoccupied with similar suicidal ideation (Sanborn, 1971; Dolkas et al., 1971). More overt suicide attempts may involve firearms, rope, knives, leaping from high places, and intentional drug overdose. Death is most often produced by a gun or rope, and overdose is most frequently associated with the unsuccessful attempt.

Concepts of Etiology. Self-destructive acts may derive from a variety of different factors, operating separately or together. Beall (1969), reviewing the literature, delineates two major etiological themes, not necessarily mutually exclusive: sociological and psychological.

From a sociological standpoint, Durkeim points out the destructive effects of rootlessness. Shore, et al. (1972), studying the Blackfoot Indians, and Ling, et al. (1970), describing suicide among post World War II Japanese youth, cite the noxiousness of cultural value breakdown and transition. Psychoanalytic writers stress the importance of such psychological factors as the inability to express anger, the actual loss or danger of loss of a loved one, and the presence of unresolved dependency and ambivalence (Beall, 1969; Toolan, 1969).

From a behavioral standpoint, Shore, et al. (1972) point out that suicide may be learned behavior and Kraus (1972) considers the presence of suicide in the family of prognostic significance.

Precipitating Stresses. Closely associated with adolescent suicide are the following stressful situations:

1. Conflict with parents
2. Academic failure
3. Frustration in love
4. Pregnancy
5. Compulsory military service (Otto, 1969)
6. Coerced therapeutic abortion in early adolescence (Copeland).

Premonitory Signs. Otto was not able to detect a specific pattern of presuicidal behavior. Instead, he noted a variety of several nonpathognomonic signs of stress which included restlessness, insomnia, irritability, hypersensitivity, nonconformity in work or at school, disregard for personal appearance, and overuse of drugs, as well as frank depressiveness or anxiety. These signs of stress did not always accompany demonstrable suicidal ideations.

Associated Diagnoses. Young people who attempt to harm themselves do not fall under one diagnostic category. Rostov (1970) describes four groups of suicidal adolescents:

1. Impulsive character disorders
2. Depressives
3. Psychotics
4. Wrist slashers

Otto (1969) similarly finds suicidal behavior in patients of varied diagnoses: neurosis, mental subnormality, depression and schizophrenia.

Despite the close relationship between suicide and depression in the adult population, this is not necessarily so for adolescents. Masterson (1970) sees self-destructive behavior more closely associated with schizophrenia than depression, and Winn notes auditory hallucinations with suicidal content in 83 percent of his adolescent inpatients.

Toolan (1969) notes, however, that adolescent depression may be frequently masked and cites a number of behavioral equivalents: boredom, the quest for sensory stimulation, restlessness, poor concentration and hypochondriasis.

Prognosis. By virtue of the multiple causes of suicide attempt, it is difficult to assess prognosis. As a rule of thumb, all attempts must be viewed as serious and treated accordingly. The following factors appear to be associated with poor prognosis.

1. A family history of suicide
2. Loss of someone important
3. A persistent theme of reunification through death with the deceased
4. Repeated attempts

The prognostic significance of suicidal behavior coexisting with schizophrenia is unclear. While Kraus finds such patients of grave concern, Winn's patients apparently did well. Further study seems warranted.

Therapeutic Considerations. Adolescent suicidal behavior may be impulsive and without dramatic forewarnings. Thus, the clinician must be on the alert for a history of suicide-evoking stresses and the presence of self-destructive tendencies. Suicidal ideation and attempts must be viewed seriously and responded to dramatically. It is far better to err on the side of conservatism than to allow a suicide that might have been prevented.

Mobilization of appropriate resources is mandatory. The therapist must actively elicit all available aids. Family members or friends must be alerted for support and surveillance of the patient. If adequate supervision cannot be guaranteed for the young patient in suicidal crisis, then hospitalization should be instituted. Strong motivation to die is another clear and obvious indication for hospitalization.

The therapist's task is to try to elicit the aid and cooperation of the suicidal adolescent's healthy ego. The therapist must take the declared position that suicide represents a poor solution to the problems at hand, that better solutions exist, and that the therapist will commit himself to help work out such solutions with the patient. External stresses must be defined and removed, if possible. Therapeutic optimism is important as well as ready availability of the therapist at all times during the crisis.

Case. June, a seventeen-year-old entering freshman, began therapy upon arriving at school. She was continuing treatment she had started with a psychiatrist at home because she was anxious and because her mother was concerned about June's isolation, bizarreness, and her obsessive interest in her father who had died four years before.

Therapy proceeded satisfactorily though unspectacularly until her mother decided to separate from her own family influence and move to another location. Upon June's return from a weekend at home, her behavior was quite bizarre and she spoke constantly of wishing to rejoin her father, as if he lived in the next town. Drowning was the intended mode of suicide although she stripped the act totally of any self-destructive significance. She was simply going to join her father. A twenty-four hour renewable anti-suicide pledge was elicited from June with the promise that the therapist would help her if she called. The Dean of Students, as well as June's mother, were alerted to the suicidal danger and June was attended constantly during the crisis. When the suicidal threat abated, psychotherapy explored connections between the lost father, the loss of extended family via mother's move and her wish to die. Thus, one particular suicidal crisis was favorably resolved, and without the need for hospitalization. Mobilization of all existing resources, however, was essential.

Psychogenic Accidents

Accidents or injurious events ostensibly caused by chance factors may be psychologically rooted in some cases (Toolan, 1969). Selzer et al. (1968) found a high incidence of psychopathy and social stress among drivers involved in multiple serious accidents. Psychogenic accidents include auto accidents or accidental drug overdoses, and may be suspected where there is a history of traumas preceded by significant emotional stress.

From a therapeutic standpoint the possible relationship between stress and accident should be noted. Destructive behavior should be regarded as poor quality problem-solving behavior by the therapist whose task would be to help develop more effective methods. Therapeutic optimism that a better way can be found is helpful. The concept of psychogenic accidents is still relatively unexplored and represents an interesting area of research.

Homicidal Behavior

Adolescents who kill, but who are not members of violent gangs, fall into the following diagnostic categories:
1. Acute schizophrenia
2. Chronic organic brain syndrome
3. Paranoid personality
4. Antisocial personality with poor impulse control

Drug or alcohol intoxication may be associated with the homicide. A history of parental seductiveness and/or brutality is not uncommon, and episodes of cruelty to animals are associated as well (MacDonald, 1967). Female adolescent murderesses may show identificational confusion and construe their violence as manifestations of masculinity (Smith, 1965).

Heterosexual Behavior Disturbance

Description

This involves sexual activity borne of emotional disorder and conflict rather than the usual developmental and cultural forces influencing the adolescent (Biele, 1971).

Nonpathological Factors Influencing Sexual Behavior

1. *Biochronology* — The form that heterosexual activity takes is a function of biological forces as well as the age of the adolescent (Caplan and Lebovici, 1969). Sexuality in early adolescence is characterized by exploration, masturbation, and in the later teens, by more serious petting and sexual intercourse (Gaguan, Beall, 1969).

2. *Culture* — There is little doubt that mores regarding sexual behavior have changed in the last two decades, resulting in a higher incidence of sexual intercourse among youth (Babikian, Caplan and Lebovici, 1969). The impact this will have upon later

heterosexual adjustment and marriage is difficult to assess.

3. *Gender* – Gender differences are evident in adolescent sexuality. Young males achieve their orgastic peaks in their late teens and early twenties (Kinsey, Pomeroy and Martin, 1948). While the drive for orgasm is intense in the male, female sexuality is more related to love and tenderness (Sherman, 1972), a drive for procreation, and the enhanced status of motherhood at this phase (Cumberlow Lodge, 1968; Biele, 1971; Babikian).

Heterosexual Disturbances

1. *Withdrawal-asceticism* – In response to newly arising, urgent and aggressive sexual feelings, some young people defend themselves against the fear of loss of control by the mechanisms of denial, repression and reaction formation. They withdraw from the opposite sex and may even develop counter-feelings of disgust. Such withdrawal and rejection of sexuality is often fluctuant, inconsistent and superficial. Occasional forays into heterosexual activity may evoke anxiety, guilt and further withdrawal (Sklansky, 1969).

With a sufficiently healthy ego, support from significant adults and peers, and the passage of time, the adolescent grows to accept sexual urges more readily and the defensive position of withdrawal-asceticism is abandoned.

Withdrawal-asceticism is to be differentiated from simple schizophrenia on the basis of its transitory nature, the retention of strong and appropriate affect, and the awareness that something is wrong.

2. *Promiscuity and prostitution* – While sexual intercourse is much more prevalent among youth, it is usually monogamous in form, producing semi-stable coupling (Caplan and Lebovici, 1969). Promiscuity, on the other hand, seems more closely associated with psychological disorder and less closely with a subcultural norm.

Promiscuous girls, studied at Cumberlow Lodge, showed a high incidence of depression, came from fatherless homes, and were frequently involved in a psychopathological mother-daughter relationship. Babikian's group of girls had personality disorders and frequent histories of developmental trauma. Russell (1971), studying a group of teenage prostitutes, found widespread maternal deprivation, a poverty of social skills, and submissiveness.

Thus, promiscuity and prostitution may be considered a heterosexual disturbance until proven otherwise in the adolescent girl. Further study is required both for male and female adolescents.

3. *Psychopathological pregnancy* – The higher incidence of sexual intercourse among teenagers parallels a higher pregnancy rate. In 1965, adolescent girls gave birth to 130,000 babies, which represented 50 percent of all out-of-wedlock births (Caplan and Lebovici, 1969). Between 1940 and 1968, the adolescent out-of-wedlock pregnancy rate increased ten-fold, from 42/1000 to 430/1000 (Babikian). Since 1967, the number of babies born to unmarried teenagers has increased at the rate of 4000 per year (Ball, 1971).

Teenage pregnancy may be categorized as follows:
   a. Nonpathological: related to curiosity, inexperience and maternal interest.
   b. Culturally related: where out-of-wedlock, teenage pregnancy and birth is reflective of a subcultural norm.
   c. Psychopathological: where pregnancy is clearly reflective of emotional problems and psychological disorder.

Naiveté and a lack of sophistication may play an important role. Perez-Reyes and Falk (1971) noted that 40 percent of the pregnant girls they studied had had sexual intercourse only one time.

The psychodynamics of adolescent pregnancy apparently vary according to social class. While sexual experimentation and neurotic conflict was noteworthy among Gagnon, Simon and Berger's (1970) group of middle-class girls, Friedman (1972) found emotional deprivation and failure of personality development common among girls coming from lower socioeconomic levels. Babikian's group of black and Puerto Rican adolescents showed a 95 percent rate of repeat pregnancies, while the London girls studied at Cumberlow Lodge demonstrated a 30 percent rate.

Individual factors associated with teenage pregnancy are family breakup, a history of maternal deprivation, and the position of oldest sibling in the family.

Diagnosis of psychopathological pregnancy can be based on the diagnosis of serious parallel psychiatric illness, a history of parental deprivation, and an intense and pathological relationship with one or both parents. From a therapeutic standpoint, psychopathological pregnancy should be viewed as premature rather than wrong. Motivation for the pregnancy should be determined. It must be pointed out that the attempt to solve problems of rejection and neglect via the birth of a child can provide only temporary relief at best. Gratification of incestuous or vengeful wishes, if present, are ultimately destructive; this too must be pointed out.

On the other hand, the achievement of the status of woman and potential mother via pregnancy may be viewed as an important accomplishment for the girl, deserving of recognition and respect. But the actual child-bearing must be taught as something to be postponed until circumstances are right both for the child as well as the mother. Psychopathological pregnancy may require family therapy or relocation of the pregnant girl to a more nurturing domicile.

With regards to the vicissitude of the actual pregnancy, several options are available: termination via therapeutic abortion, delivery and placement, and motherhood for the adolescent girl. Occasionally a teenager insists upon her rights to bear her child and raise it despite psychiatric advice to the contrary. In the face of parental ambivalence or indecisiveness, this poses a difficult therapeutic problem. Forced interruption of the pregnancy in the absence of psychosis is probably antitherapeutic and may be illegal. Much postpartum support both for the mother and child is indicated in this difficult situation. A therapeutic abortion that is coerced may result in depression and suicidal behavior. The insistence upon abortion by a parent who is already considered as rejecting by the teenager may constitute the ultimate rejection (Senay, 1970).

In the presence of psychological support, realistic plans for further education and development and an optimistic view of the future, the actual choice between therapeutic abortion, or postpartum placement may be simply a matter of expediency.

Therapeutic abortion may be indicated for those girls impregnated through inexperience and more interested in continuing their education than in motherhood. (Perez-Reyes and Falk, 1971).

4. *Male sexual dysfunction* — With the higher involvement of adolescent males in sexual intercourse, sexual problems such as failure to have an erection and premature ejaculation have been reported.

From an etiological standpoint, true impotency and premature ejaculation are usually associated with a number of neurotic conflicts, including those of maternal dependency, masculine identification, and incestuousness in the older adolescent and young adult. In addition, sexual dysfunction may reflect a more serious failure of personality development. On the other hand, it may simply indicate the intense anxiety of the inexperienced young male.

From the therapeutic standpoint, reduction of this anxiety represents the initial task of treatment.

5. *Drugs and sex* — A variety of drugs have been used by young people in quest of greater orgastic pleasure. Amyl nitrate, alcohol, doxipine and other chemical agents have been reported to have aphrodesiac properties; but it is uncertain how much of the sexual enhancement is pharmacological in nature and how much is attributable to the psychology of the hosts. Dosage seems to be an important variable in this connection. At higher levels, drugs taken for aphrodesiac effects often suppress sexuality. The impotency of the heroin addict is one example.

Pharmacopathia (Drug Misuse)

Description

Drug misuse is a psychophysiological disturbance resulting from heavy and often uncontrolled use of certain pharmacological agents in individuals with underlying psychopathology.

Epidemiology and Cultural Considerations

The development and use of drugs for medicinal effects is one of the hallmarks of our modern culture. Their use for purposes other than the correction of physical illness is relatively new. With the development of psychotropic drugs, much impetus was given to the practice of using chemical agents for psychological purposes. Now the extra-medical use of mind-altering drugs is widespread and with it has come a misuse that is of epidemic proportions. Revised statistics on drug consumption reappear with great frequency and continue to show an upward trend. The office of Drug Abuse Law Enforcement, as of April, 1972, reported about 500,000 heroin addicts and twenty million marijuana and hashish users in the United States (Gaukler, 1972).

Heroin addicts are located principally in larger cities with New York City as the current mecca. Heroin is found to a lesser degree in suburbia and least of all in rural areas. Approximately one in two opiate users is black and one in four is Spanish speaking. Most are males between the ages of 18 and 25 (Adler, unpublished). Users of cannabis derivatives (marijuana and hashish) are ubiquitous and are found in larger cities, small towns, and in the ghetto, as well as on the college campus. Cannabis is used by physicians (Lipp and Benson, 1972), as well as seventh graders (Larimer, 1971).

There is much evidence indicating that users of one drug have access to a number of other drugs as well and most probably use them to differing degrees. The concept that "soft drugs" (cannabis derivatives) do not lead to "hard drugs" (opiates) is simplistic and misrepresentative. Individuals able to obtain one drug are exposed to a variety of others, including narcotics. Individuals with underlying personality problems, thus exposed, are candidates for addiction (Gaukler, 1972). The opportunity to experiment with addictive drugs on the part of a susceptible host are the two essential ingredients for drug addiction.

Patterns of Drug Use

First use of chemical agents for psychological effects usually occurs around puberty and takes the form of beer and wine-drinking, glue-sniffing, and marijuana and hashish smoking. Adolescents wishing to go beyond superficial experimentation have ready access to a variety of drugs via contact with older adolescents and a certain number of them do (Butzer, 1972). Heavy users of marijuana and hashish are especially prone to using other drugs, and heavy use is positively correlated with significant pre-existing psychopathology on the part of the host (Little, 1972).

Certain drugs such as cannabis have wide appeal and are constantly sought, while others, such as LSD, are in vogue one year and passé the next. Cocaine and methqualone (Quaalude ®) are current favorites (Lipinski, 1972).

How a drug is used appears to be influenced by three factors:

1. The host, his state of mind and mental health
2. The supply and popularity of a particular chemical agent
3. The value-systems of a society and its significant subcultures (Lipinski, 1972).

Classification of Drug Users

In the contemporary American society drug users may be categorized as follows:

1. *Experimental users.* Large numbers of the adolescent population fall into this category, but only a small percentage regularize the use of drugs. With regard to cannabis, of the estimated 24 million Americans who have used it only about 2 percent have become heavy users (Gaukler, 1972). This group of experimental users requires little psychiatric care or general concern.

2. *Controlled users.* This group uses one or more drugs in a controlled manner with no apparent impairment of function or adaptation and with perhaps a greater feeling of immediate well-being as a consequence. In this category is found large segments of the population who ingest, with or without medical prescription, a great variety of chemically active ingredients ranging from tranquilizers to alcohol to cannabis.

With regard to youth and the controlled use of drugs, it should be noted that:

a. Adolescence is not characterized as a period of moderation and self-control.
b. The younger the adolescent, the less likely he is to control the use of drugs once he has become involved.

    c. Personality breakdown may be the first clue to a pre-existing emotional disorder unmasked by drugs, and repair of coexisting psychological and physiological problems is therapeutically most difficult (Little, 1972).

    d. Knowledge of the long-term effects of chemical agents upon the special physiology of the adolescent has not been established.

Thus, while large segments of the population use drugs in a controlled fashion, the evidence of misuse is probably greatest among adolescents.

3. *Pharmacopaths.* It has been estimated that 2 percent of the youth group smoking hashish and marijuana are heavy users (Gaukler, 1972) and have a high incidence of psychopathology (Rosenberg and Patch, 1972). Their use of drugs is often uncontrolled and accompanied by a breakdown of personality functions.

Treatment is difficult as there is the two-fold task of dealing with the drug-induced physiological problem on the one hand as well as with the underlying psychological problem on the other (Little, 1972). Yet this group of young people must number in the hundreds of thousands.

Pathological drug users may start with alcohol, progress to barbituates and amphetamines, and then get involved with opiates (Frederick, 1972).

From a diagnostic standpoint, the pharmacopath may be neurotic, schizophrenic or manifest a personality disorder. He is frequently depressed and suicidal (Dolkart, et al., 1971; Sanborn, 1971).

Complications arising from the pathological use of drugs are academic failure, personality breakdown, a variety of adverse side effects from impurities and drug mixtures, idiosyncratic reactions, overdosage, and withdrawal reactions (Papavasiliou, 1972).

The overall death rate in this young drug population is considerably higher than that of the statistical average. Aside from other forms of death (Beall, 1969), the suicidal rate is three times that of the general population and the homicidal rate is 25 times as great in this drug using group.

Treatment and rehabilitation have been largely unsuccessful to date. The use of methadone for heroin addicts is of limited value for adolescents. The development of a multimodality treatment approach including a drug-free, sheltered environment, may be a fruitful avenue of exploration.

Major Drugs Used

While drug vogues vary with the times, six groups have been used frequently and consistently:
1. Cannabis sativa derivatives (marijuana and hashish)
2. Major hallucinogens (e.g. Lysergic Acid)
3. Stimulants (amphetamines and cocaine)
4. Depressants (barbiturates and volatile solvents)
5. Opiates

While the following drugs will be presented in terms of their effects, it must be remembered that the total impact is multidetermined and influenced by the host, the chemical agent, and the social context (Cannabis, 1968).

Cannabis Sativa Derivatives

Description. Cannabis sativa is the generic name for Indian hemp. The dried leaves are called marijuana and the resin obtained from the flowering tops is called hashish. The active ingredient isolated thus far is tetrahydrocannabinal or THC. It is considered a minor hallucinogen (Cannabis, 1968). Common names are: stick, "j", joint, pot, dope, grass (marijuana), hash (hashish).

Mode of Use. Smoked, occasionally drunk as "tea," or sniffed.

Clinical Features:

Odor:	Burned leaves, rope
Autonomic signs and signs	Increased pulse, blood pressure and deep tendon reflexes.
Eyes:	Conjunctival injection, photo-sensitivity
Mood:	Elated or "high"
Behavior:	Giggly, loud and excessive speech, ataxia
Perceptions:	Heightened and perhaps distorted (Cannabis is a minor hallucinogen)

Appetite: Increased, especially for sweets (Ball,
                             Chambers and Ball, 1968, Cannabis,
                             1968)
Duration: One to six hours

Adverse Side Effects — (Associated with heavy use or two
cigarettes or more per session (Louria and Wolfson, 1972).

1. "Amotivational syndrome" or breakdown of personality
   function and arrest of psychological development.
2. Psychological dependence
3. Pharyngitis, bronchitis
4. Acute toxic psychosis (Talbott and Teague, 1969; Farnsworth, 1972; Louria and Wolfson, 1972).

Research into the long-term effects of Cannabis sativa is
incomplete. The possible use of Cannabis for therapeutic purpose
is just being investigated.

Treatment. Probably no medication is required for the acute
toxic phase which may last from one hour to several days,
depending on the amount taken (Talbott and Teague, 1969).
Chlorpromazine may be prescribed for anxiety or paranoid
ideation. Amotivation syndrome and psychological dependence
may be associated with serious psychological problems requiring
psychiatric intervention.

Major Hallucinogens

Description. A heterogeneous family of drugs that distort and
intensify sensory perceptions. They may produce visual hallucinations, suggestibility, and personality fragmentation.

Types.
1. *LSD* (lysergic acid diethylamide)
   Common names: Acid, sugar, Big D, cubes.
2. *Psilocibin* (3 — 2 dimethylamino) Ethylindol — 4 —
   dihydrogen Phosphate)
   Common names: Mushroom
3. *Mescaline* (3, 4, 5 trimethoxy phenylethylamine; alcaloid
   from Peyote)
   Common names: cactus, peyote
4. *DMT* (Di methyltryptamine)
   Common names: Businessman's high

5. *DOM* (3 Methoxy — 4, 5 Methylene Dioxy Amphetamine)
Common names: STP or security, tranquility and peace.

Modes of Use. DMT may be smoked with tobacco and the others are swallowed.

Clinical Features

Eyes:	Mydriasis (dilated pupils)
Palms:	Cold and sweaty
Behavior:	Preoccupation with perceptions, "into things."
Mood;	Exhilarated
Thinking:	Suggestible
Companion:	Often present
Duration:	From one hour (DMT) to one to three days (DOM, high dosage). An LSD "trip" may last from eight to twelve hours.

Adverse Side Effects (LSD)

1. Bad Trip:	Experience of panic or paranoid delusions.
2. Acute organic brain syndrome:	Anxiety, decreased memory, confusion, disorientation
3. "Flashbacks":	The recurrence of symptoms and sensations from previous ingestion.

4. Amotivational syndrome and personality breakdown.
5. Accidental trauma from misperceptions.

In addition there have been reports of chromosomal damage and suicide associated with use of LSD (Louria and Wolfson, 1972). LSD may produce agitation and such atropine effects as dry mouth and difficulty in breathing and swallowing. Administration of phenothiazines may augment these untoward side effects.

Treatment. The "bad trip" may be alleviated by suggestion and psychological support. Panic may be controlled by phenothiazines and barbiturates. Latent emotional disorders unmasked by, the hallucinogens may require psychiatric intervention. Anxiety, paranoia, confusion and disorientation may abate in time.

Stimulants

Included in this group are the amphetamines (dextroamphetamine, methamphetamine) and cocaine (Benzo-methylecgonine).

1. *Amphetamines*

Mode of use: Swallowed or injected.

Clinical Features:

Mood	Exuberant — "high"
Behavior	Excited, energetic, restless
Insomnia	
Anorexia	
Tremor	
Skin	Sweating
Tachycardia	
Needle marks	
Urine test (methylorange): positive	
Duration:	Four hours

Adverse side effects and complications.

Physical tolerance with need for increasing doses

Psychological dependency

Psychosis resembling paranoid schizophrenia

Acute organic brain syndrome

Rebound depression and suicide

Vascular hypertension

Intracranial hemorrhage

Infections — cellulitis, hepatitis, endocarditis

Malnutrition

Arrythmias

Treatment. Phenothiazines may be used to calm excitement and anxiety. Psychiatric and general medical attention may be required for the other complications.

2. *Cocaine*

Mode of Use: Sniffed, injected or swallowed

Clinical Features: Intense euphoria, restlessness, hyper-activity, rapid pulse, hyperactive reflexes

Duration: Fifteen to thirty minutes of euphoria

Adverse Side Effects and Complications

Psychological dependence

Perforation of nasal septum

Paranoid reactions

Amotivational syndrome and personality breakdown
Anorexia and malnutrition
Overdose: Preconvulsive with muscle twitchings
Withdrawal: Depression and suicide.
Treatment:
Barbiturates for convulsion
Respiratory depression: Physiological support
Psychological Depression: Psychiatric intervention

Depressants

Depressants constitute a large and heterogeneous group of chemical agents which depress the central nervous system, producing stupor after an initial period of well-being. Included in this group are the barbiturates, volatile solvents, and the opiate derivatives. The opiate group will be considered separately.

1. *Barbiturates*
   Included are phenobarbital, amobarbital, pentobarbital, secobarbital.
   Common names: Downs, barbs, goofballs, blue heavens, yellow jacket, red devils

Mode of use. Swallowed or injected.
Clinical Features

Behavior: Calm, drowsy or drunken without smell of alcohol.
Vital signs: (Pulse, respiration) decreased.
Urine: Positive
Positive pentobarbital test reaction: .2 gm produces no clinical effects of calm or drowsiness in two hours.
Duration: Four hours or longer
Adverse Side Effects
Physical tolerance
Physical withdrawal: Convulsions
Overdosage: Death via central nervous system depression
Amotivational Syndrome with personality breakdown.
Treatment. Physical tolerance requires gradual withdrawal with pentobarbital or chlordiazepoxide. Overdosage requires physiological support. Amotivational syndrome requires psychiatric

intervention and rehabilitation.

2. *Volatile Solvents (Glue sniffing)*

Contained in this group are carbon tetrachloride, acetone, benzine, toluene, acetone n-hexane and other chemical agents found in glue, cleaning fluids, deodorants, etc.

Mode of Use. These volatile solvents contained in glue and other chemical agents are sniffed.

Clinical features:

Behavior: Excitation, then stupor; impaired judgment and co-ordination.

Mood: Delusions, euphoria, then depression, slurred speech.

Duration: Two hours

Adverse Side Effects and Complications.

Cardiac arrythmia and death (associated with physical exertion)

Renal and hepatic dysfunction

Bone marrow depression

Organic brain syndrome

Polyneuropathy

Treatment.

Symptomatic

Opiate Derivitives

Description:

Heroin (diacytyl morphine), morphine sulfate and methadone (methadone hyprochloride) are the most common members of the opiate family implicated in drug abuse.

Common names: Heroin – H, horse, junk, scag and smack.
                    Morphine – Dreamer
                    Methadone – Dolly

Mode of use. Heroin is sniffed, injected subcutaneously (skin popped), and injected intravenously (mainlined).

Methadone and morphine are swallowed or injected.

Clinical features – Heroin

Behavior: Drowsiness and nodding post injection.

Mood: Serenity, then sleep

Pupils: Pinpoint

Pulse: Slow

Respiration: Slow
Skin: Needle marks
Appetite: For sweets
Methadone produces similar features to heroin with less sedation and somnolence.
Duration: Heroin — Four hours
Adverse Side Effects and Complications — Heroin
Overdose: Respiratory depression
       Cardiac arrythmia
       Pulmonary edema
       Coma and death

Physical tolerance
Psychological dependence
Withdrawal symptoms:
 After eight hours — Autonomic symptoms: mydriasis, rhinorrhea, yawning, chills
 After five to ten days: Nausea, vomiting, diarrhea, twitching, "gooseflesh," pain in abdomen and muscles
        Serum hepatitus
        Tetanus
        Neurologic abnormalities
        Renal dysfunction

Treatment
Overdose: (Respiratory depression):
       Antagonists (nalorphine)
       Stimulants (caffeine and sodium benzoate)
       Artificial respiration
Withdrawal: Heroin and methadone in tapering doses.
Physical
Complications: Hospitalization
Drug free therapeutic communities such as Synanon may be helpful for rehabilitation.

Methadone use may produce the same problems of withdrawal, respiratory depression, and pulmonary edema; treatment should be geared accordingly.

Schizophrenoid Disturbance (Boyer, 1971)

Description

A syndrome occurring in adolescence characterized by disturbances in thinking, mood and behavior resembling schizophrenia. It is differentiated from schizophrenia by virtue of dramatic remissions that may occur, by virtue of etiological factors associated with the adolescent disturbance not usually associated with schizophrenia (e.g. amphetamine-induced "paranoid schizophrenia") and by virtue of the clinician's need to not stigmatize adolescents with the poor prognosis associated with schizophrenia.

Schizophrenoid disturbance may appear as an acute schizophrenic episode described in DSM II or may present a less florid form characterized by withdrawal and absence of affect.

Etiologically, a schizophrenoid disturbance may be drug-induced (as with the amphetamines), infectious (encephalitis) (Carboz, 1969), or ideopathic. Constitutional and family stresses are no doubt present to varying degrees along with the phase-specific stresses of adolescence.

Schizophrenoid disturbance of adolescence may be differentiated from schizophrenia on the basis of a careful history (drugs, infections), a dramatic remission in the face of a vigorous psychotherapeutic intervention, and the preservation of a reality sense, affect and human relatedness in the face of florid symptoms. Projective testing may be helpful.

Therapy may require a multi-faceted approach including hospitalization, detoxification, individual psychotherapy, and family therapy as well as educative and rehabilitative help (Carboz, 1969; Boyer, 1971). The sooner and more vigorous the therapeutic intervention, the greater likelihood of success.

Psychosocial Disturbances

Description

A heterogeneous group of disturbances of behavior, affect and thinking related to psychological and social stresses. They include

1. Family unit disturbance
2. Alienation disturbance
3. Minor group delinquent disturbance
4. Runaway disturbance
5. Pharmacopathia

Runaway disturbance has been described under flight-behavior disturbance for purposes of convenience; pharmacopathia has been described separately due to the extensiveness of the subject, although it will be considered a psychosocial disturbance.

Family Unit Disturbance

Description

This is disturbed behavior, thinking, and affect more reflective of a psychopathological family interactional system than an intrapsychic conflict within the adolescent (Ackerman, 1970; Redl and Wineman, 1951; Shapiro, 1972).

Discovery of family pathology often comes about through evaluation of the adolescent who is presented for treatment but who serves as the bridge to treatment for other family members.

Family stress may be qualitative, e.g. double bind, covert hostility, or quantitative in which rejection, neglect or absence may be operant. A therapeutic approach should include careful evaluation of the family dynamics so that family therapy, individual therapy and other modalities employed can be most effective.

Alienation Disturbance (The "Hippy")

Description

A pattern of behavior and associated values characterized by:
1. Rejection of official cultural standards such as industry, cleanliness, "success," respect for authority and formal education.
2. Withdrawal from societally-approved fields of activity such as school, work or military service.

3. Adherence to a subculture value system often characterized by a dress code (e.g. jeans, long hair, lack of personal grooming), the use of drugs, freer sexual attitudes, communal living, disinterest in traditional work and advancement, and a pacifistic orientation. It is considered pathological when ego functions and psychological development cease as a consequence.

Alienation is to be differentiated from the Minor Group Delinquent Reaction which is less interested in social protest and more involved with petty stealing and gang activities; it may be also differentiated from the rebellious counter-cultures (e.g. Yippy) which are more politically activist and violence-oriented. It is also to be differentiated from the usual adolescent quest for separateness. It may be differentiated from a schizophrenoid disturbance by the absence of bizarreness and withdrawal.

The etiology of alienation disturbance is multiple and probably reflective of unusual sociocultural stresses which, coupled with the usual developmental difficulties of adolescence, produce the default phenomenon of alienation.

With regard to treatment, many of the alienated young people who have mental illness are psychologically supported by their peers and need no therapeutic intervention. When treatment is rendered, the clinician must always be cognizant of and respect operant subcultural values.

Many hippys later return to society's matrix as they become older, to again pursue lives more adaptive to society and more commensurate with their new chronological status of adult.

Prognosis is best determined by the number of positive accomplishments, the degree of family support, the amount of damage due to drugs, and the degree of pre-existing psychopathology.

Again, it should be noted that alienation disturbance is not a mental illness per se but a reaction to the stresses of current society.

Minor Group Delinquent Disturbance

Individuals with this psychosocial disorder have acquired the values and behavior of a delinquent peer group or gang to whom they are loyal and with whom they characteristically steal, truant, and absent themselves from home for varying periods of time. They are often sexually active (Ulmar, 1970; Jenkins, 1971; DSM II, 1968).

Female counterparts may become "auxiliary" members of the boys' gang or, more rarely, may form a gang of their own.

Etiologically, it should be noted that peer grouping is a normal function of adolescence and important in the process of separating from parents and establishing autonomy. A broken home or devitalized family may foster antisocial gang formation as well, just as the urban ghetto does with its turbulence and insularity.

Treatment of minor delinquency is probably best accomplished through channelization of the entire gang into active and constructive programs, job training, and the employment of youth workers for purposes of direction and identification.

The minor group delinquent disturbance is to be differentiated from the violent group delinquent disturbance by the absence of violence, territoriality and a history of multiple arrests.

Psychophysiological Disturbances

Description

A group of multietiological body disorders occurring in adolescence in which the psychological component is of considerable importance. The predisposition for a psychophysiological disturbance may be covert at this phase only to become more manifest at a later date (Sperling).

Classification

Psychophysiological disturbances may be grouped according to the degree of somatic involvement:
1. Symptomatic: e.g. the painful headache
2. Symptomatic with physical signs: e.g. cramps and spasms of mucus colitis.
3. Syndromes: e.g. ulcerative colitis with symptoms, signs as well as tissue changes (Szasz, 1952).

Grouping may be according to severity:
1. Degree of precipitating stress
2. Degree of pain
3. Degree of dysfunction of organ system and personality
4. Degree of tissue change
5. Degree of psychological symptoms

With evaluation of the above factors, severity may be described in terms of mild, moderate or marked.

Some of the more common psychophysiological disturbances noted in adolescence are anorexia nervosa, obesity, asthma, enuresis, ulcerative colitis, headaches, hypertension, allergy, and regional enteritis (Finch, 1972; Heath, 1968; McCaffery, 1970).

Pseudocyesis, peptic ulcer, eczema, angioneurotic edema and migraine have also been noted (Barglow, 1969).

Anorexia Nervosa (Dyspepsia Hysterica)

Description

This is a psychophysiological eating disturbance occurring mostly in girls, beginning at puberty and characterized by disinterest in and abstinence from food. There is an associated weight loss of twenty-five pounds or more (Blaine, 1971). The incidence of anorexia nervosa is 50-75/100,000 with a mortality rate greater than 15 percent. While this is chiefly a disorder of pubescent girls, Blaine reports an 11 percent incidence among boys.

Bruch (1970) classifies anorexia nervosa into primary, or related to a body image disturbance, and secondary, related to another psychological problem.

Jochmus (1967) notes gender-specific differences in the under-lying psychodynamics with mother fixation important for girls and problems of self-esteem noteworthy among boys. Blaine finds other dynamic factors associated including pregnancy phantasies, anger at the family and feelings of rejection.

Symptoms include not only refusal to eat but also hiding of food, bulemia with formed vomit and later, emaciation, depressiveness, constipation and apathy (Jochmus, 1967; Blaine, 1971).

The disturbance may be triggered by a precipitating stress in the form of an accusation or a crisis of guilt.

Therapy may have to be lifesaving and heroic and include tube feeding and intravenous infusions. While many psychotherapeutic approaches have been tried, none has been proven more effective than others (Blaine, 1971).

This condition is to be differentiated from an underlying schizophrenia (Finch, 1971).

Obesity

Description

Obesity is enlarged body size due to excessive accumulation of fat tissue; it is rooted in both constitutional and psychological disorders. It is associated with a variety of psychiatric disorders or with no psychopathology at all (Bruch, 1970).

Prognostically, less than one third of a group of obese adolescents studied outgrew obesity. Many of those who remained frankly obese after adolescence manifested serious concomitant mental problems (Finch). Body concept, self-image, and the symbolic use of food are important mechanisms in the development of obesity, especially in adolescents, whose anatomies and physiologies are in great transition. The presence of obesity in one or both parents is also important.

Finch sees many obese adolescents as essentially depressive, with a history of maternal deprivation and who develop anxiety in association with the eating process. Identification with an obese parent is also of major dynamic significance.

Treatment must hinge not only upon insight into early developmental trauma but also on repair of body image, diet control, exercise habits, and correction of pathological child-parent relationships (Bruch, 1971).

Prognosis is determined by the overall pattern of personality developments and strengths.

Headache

Psychophysiological headaches are associated with such factors as introspectiveness, repression (Heath, 1968), depression (Ling, et al., 1970), and anxiety; and therapy must be geared accordingly.

Ulcerative colitis

This is a multietiological illness of the lower bowel character- ized by cramps, diarrhea with the passage of blood and mucus as well as pathological changes in the tissue of the large bowel. Eventual nutritional and electrolyte imbalance may occur. It may assume an acute or chronic form, and perforation and exsangui- nation may occur in acute cases.

From a psychological point of view, adolescents with ulcerative colitis fall under a number of diagnoses including depression, passive-dependency, obsessive-compulsive neurosis, and with- drawal (McCaffery, 1970).

Characterologically, adolescent colitis may be classified as
1. Pseudomature, where obsessive "little men and women" may develop symptoms at times of change in the life styles.
2. Adolescents with passive-aggressive, manipulative traits.

Treatment requires a combined approach which may include a psychiatrist, an internist and a surgeon. Psychotherapy may decrease mortality but not the incidence of surgery (Finch).

Asthma

When asthma is accompanied by allergy, psychological problems are of secondary importance. Separation of the asthmatic adoles- cent from his family may reduce the incidence of attacks (Finch).

Enuresis

This condition may be defined as bedwetting beyond the fifth year or the time of maturation of bladder control. It is often chronic and persistent from childhood and may be primary, with the adolescent perpetually wet. While a certain number may have organic pathology, it is rarely considered the sole causative factor. On the other hand, most enuretics manifest considerable social and psychological pathology (Murphy and Chapman, 1970).

Psychodynamically, fear of genital injury and confusion about body image are important (DeLuca, 1968).

Treatment should include urological evaluation; psychotherapy should foster increased self-controls as well as correction of destructive phantasies. Family cooperation is often essential.

BIBLIOGRAPHY

Ackerman, N.: Family psychotherapy today. Family Process, 9: 123-126, 1970.

Adam and Eve: Differences in biology. M.D., May, 1972, pp. 89-91.

Adler, D.: The psychodynamics of adolescent opiate addiction. Unpublished.

Arietti, S.: Manic-depressive psychosis. In Arietti, S. (Ed.): American Handbook of Psychiatry. New York, Basic, 1959, vol. I, pp. 455-507.

Aronow, R., et al.: Childhood poisonings: An unfortunate consequence of methadone availability. JAMA, 219: 321-323, 1972.

Athanasiou, R.: Multiple orgasms and age. Human Sexuality, 7:11, 1973.

Baker, H., and Stoller, R.: Can a biological force contribute to gender identity? Am J Psychiatry, 124:1653, 1968.

Ball, G.: The doctor and the law: Teenage pregnancies and the law. The New Physician, 14:663, 1971.

Ball, J., Chambers, C., and Ball, M.: The association of marijuana smoking with opiate addiction in the United States. J Criminal Law, Criminology and Police Science, 59:171-182, 1968.

Balser, B., and Masterson, J.: Suicide in adolescents. Am J Psychiatry, 116:400-404, 1959.

Barglow, P.: Pseudocyesis and psychiatric sequellae of sterilization. Arch Gen Psychiatry, 11:571-580, 1969.

Beall, L.: The dynamics of suicide: A review of the literature 1897-1965. Bulletin of Suicidology, 1:2-15, 1969.

Benedek, E.: Child custody laws: Their psychiatric implications. Am J Psychiat, 129:326-328, 1972.

Beshai, J.: Behavioral correlates of the EEG in delinquents. J Psychol, 79:141-146, 1971.

Biele, A.: Unwanted pregnancy: Symptoms of depressive practice. Am J Psychiat, 128:748-760, 1971.

Blacker, K., and Wong, N.: Four cases of autocastration. Arch Gen Psychiatry, 8:169-177, 1963.

Blaine, G.: Adjustment reaction of adolescence. Psychiatric Annals, 1:46-51, 1971a

Blaine, G.: Depression and suicide. Psychiatric Annals, 1:58-67, 1971b

Borowitz, G.: Character disorders in childhood and adolescence. In Feinstein, S., Giovacchini, P., and Miller, A. L., (Eds.): Adolescent Psychiatry, New York, Basic, 1971, vol. I, pp. 343-363.

Boston Collaborative Drug Surveillance Program: Adverse drug reactions. JAMA, 219:217, 1972.

Boyer, B.: Interactions among stimulus barrier, maternal overprotective barrier, innate drive tensions and maternal overstimulation. In Feinstein, S., Giovacchini, P., and Miller, A. (Eds.): Adolescent Psychiatry. New York, Basic, 1971, vol. I, pp. 363-379.

Bruch, H.: Anorexia nervosa in the male. Psychosom Med, 33:31-47, 1971.

Bruch, H.: Eating disorders in adolescence. In Zubin, J., and Freedman, A. (Eds.): The Psychopathology of Adolescence. New York, Grune, 1970.

Butzer, S.: Covert drug abuse. JAMA, 219:1633-1634, 1972.

Campbell, D.: The electroencephalogram in cannabis-associated psychosis. Can Psychiatr Assoc J, 16:161-165, 1971.

Cannabis. Report by the Advisory Committee on Drug Dependence, Home office, London, Her Majesty's Stationery Office, 1968.

Caplan, G., and Lebovici, S.: Depression and suicide. In Caplan, G., and Lebovici, S. (Eds.): Adolescence: Psychosocial Perspectives. New York, Basic, 1969.

Carboz, R.: Endogenous psychoses of the adolescent. In Caplan, G., and Lebovici, S. (Eds.): Adolescence: Psychosocial Perspectives. New York, Basic, 1969.

Carlin, A., and Post, R.: Patterns of drug use among marijuana smokers. JAMA, 218:867-868, 1971.

Chapel, J., and Taylor, D.: Glue sniffing. Mo Med, 65:288-292, 1968.

Cheatham, J.: A profile of the drug-dependent patient. South Med J, 64:1354-1357, 1971.

Chodoff, P.: Changing styles in the neuroses. In Highlights of 125th Annual Meeting of the Amer Psychiatric Assoc, Dallas, Texas, May 1-5, 1972. Psychiatric Spectator, 7:11-14.

Chwast, J.: Socio-psychological aspects: Special problems in treating female offenders. Int J Offender Therapy, 15:24-27, 1971.

Cohen, C., et al.: Interpersonal patterns of personality for drug-abusing patients and their therapeutic implications. Arch Gen Psychiatry, 24:353-358, 1971.

Cohen, S., and Ditman, K.: Prolonged adverse reactions to lysergic acid and diethylamide. Arch Gen Psychiatry, 8:975, 1963.

Contraception for teenagers. Caplan, H., moderator. Med Aspects of Human Sexuality, Oct, 1972.

Cooper, H.: Self-mutilation by Peruvian prisoners. Int J Offender Therapy, 15:180-188, 1971

Copeland, A.: The violent black gang. To be published in Feinstein, S., Giovacchini, P., and Miller, A. (Eds.): Adolescent Psychiatry. New York, Basic, 1974, vol. 3.

Copeland, A.: The Runaway. Unpublished.

Costello, A., Gunn, J., and Dominian, J.: Etiological factors in young schizophrenic men. Br J Psychiatry, 114:433-441, 1968.

Council Report: Treatment of morphine-type dependence by withdrawal methods. JAMA, 219:1611-1615, 1972.

Council Report: Oral methodone maintenance techniques in the management of morphine-type dependence. JAMA, 219:1618-1619, 1972.

Crabtree, L., and Tasjian, L.: Drug abuse within an adolescent treatment center. Psychiatric Annals, 2:26-45, 1972.

Cramer, B.: Delusion of pregnancy in a girl with drug-induced lactation. Am J Psychiatry, 127:960-963, 1971.

Cumberlow Lodge: Aspects of Remand and Classifying. Printed by the London Borough of Lambeth, 1968.

Dalton, K.: The Premenstrual Syndrome. Springfield, Thomas, 1964.

Davidson, S.: Auto enucleation of the eye — a study of self-mutilation. Acta Psychother, 10:286-300, 1962.

DeBray, L.: Delinquency in Venezuela. Int J Offender Therapy, 15:71-73, 1968.

DeLuca, A.: Psychosocial conflict in adolescent enuretics. J Psychol, 68:145-149, 1968

Diagnostic and Statistical Manual of Mental Disorders (DSM II), Washington D.C., American Psychiatric Assoc., 1968.

Dobbs, W.: Methadone treatment of heroin addicts. JAMA, 218:1536-1541, 1971.

Dolkast, M., et al.: Suicide preoccupations in young affluent American drug users: A study of yippies at the Democratic Convention. Bulletin of Suicidology, Fall, 1971.

Douglas, J.: Youth in Turmoil: Crime and Delinquency Issues. Chevy Chase, Md., NIMH Center for Studies of Crime and Delinquency, 1970.

Drug abuse now epidemic: What's being done about it? U.S. News and World Report, April, 1972, pp. 38-45.

Drug Addiction in Israel. From Proceedings of the Symposium on Drug Addiction in Israel. Jerusalem, June 1-2, 1970. Publication of the Inst. of Criminology, No. 17, Jerusalem, 1970.

Erikson, E.: Identity and the life cycle, monograph, Psychol Issues, I: , 1959.

Erikson, E.: Womanhood and the inner space. In Identity, Youth and Crisis. New York, Norton, 1968.

Esson, W.: Symptomatic autism in childhood and adolescence. Pediatrics, 47:717-722, 1971.

Falsenberg, R.: "Unfeminine" delinquent girls. Int J Offender Therapy, 15:21-23, 1971.

Farberow, N., and Schneidman, E.: The Cry for Help. New York, McGraw, 1961.

Farnsworth, D.: Marijuana: A signal of misunderstanding. Summary of the report from the National Commission on Marijuana and Drug Abuse. Psychiatric Annals, 2:9-25, 1972.

Fein, E.: Repeat pregnancies: Learning from a demonstration project, In Highlights: 23rd Annual Meeting of the American Association of Psychiatric Services for Children, Beverly Hills, Calif., Nov. 17-21, 1971.

Finch, S.: Childhood psychophysiologic disorders. Consultant, April, 1972, pp. 163-165.

Finch, S., and Poznansky, E.: Adolescent Suicide. Springfield, Thomas, 1971.

Finkelstein, B.: Parenteral hyperalimentation in anorexia nervosa. JAMA, 219:217, 1972.

Fiumara, N.: Venereal disease. Pediatr Clin North Am, 16:333-345, 1969.

Frederick, C.: Drug abuse as self-destructive behavior. Drug Therapy, March, 1972, pp. 46-48.

Friedman, C.: Unwed mothers: A continuing problem. Am J Psychiatry, 129:85-89, 1972.

Gadpaille, W.: Innate masculine-feminine differences. Med Aspects of Human Sexuality, February, 1973.

Gagnon, J., Simon, W., and Berger, A.: Some aspects of sexual adjustment in early and later adolescence. In Zubin, J., and Freedman, A. (Eds.): The Psychopathology of Adolescence. New York, Grune, 1970.

Garmezy, N.: Vulnerable children: Implications derived from studies of an internalizing-externalizing symptom dimension. In Zubrin, J., and Freedman, A. (Eds.): The Psychopathology of Adolescence. New York, Grune, 1970.

Gaukler, R.: Present-day view of marijuana. Philadelphia Med, May, 1972, pp. 329-331.

Gay, G., and Sheppard, C.: Sex in the drug-culture. Med Aspects of Human Sexuality, October, 1972.

Gilbert, J.: Clinical Psychological Tests in the Psychiatric and Medical Practice. Springfield, Thomas, 1969.

Giovacchini, P.: Fantasy formation, ego defect and identity problems. In Feinstein, S., Giovacchini, P., and Miller, A. (Eds.): Adolescent Psychiatry. New York, Basic, 1971, vol. I.

Glaser, F.: The British system and the American system: The development of narcotic control. Philadelphia Med, May, 1972, pp. 319-325.

Glass, G., et al: Psychiatric emergency related to the menstrual cycle. Am J Psychiatry, 128:705-711, 1971.

Glossary of Terms in the Drug Culture. Bureau of Narcotics and Dangerous Drugs, U.S. Govt. Printing Office, 1971.

Goldberg, M.: Facts and myths about the homosexual patient. Consultant, March, 1972, pp. 166-169.

Gonzolez, E., and Dawney, J.: Polyneuropathy in a glue sniffer. Arch Phys Med Rehabil, 55:333-337, 1972.

Goode, E.: Drug use and sexual activity on a college campus. Am J Psychiatry, 128:1272-1276, 1972.

Goshen, C.: The characterology of adolescent offenders and the management of prisons. Reflections, 7:1-19, 1972.

Gould, R.: The case for heroin maintenance therapy. Drug Therapy, May, 1972, pp. 67-71.

Graff, H., and Mallin, R.: The syndrome of wristcutters. Am J Psychiatry, 124:36-42, 1967.

Green, A.: Self-mutilation in schizophrenic children. Arch Gen Psychiatry, 17:234-244, 1967.

Grinspoon, L., and Hedblom, P.: Amphetamine abuse. Drug Therapy, January, 1972, pp. 83-99.

Grunebaum, H., and Klerman, G.: Wrist-slashing. Am J Psychiatry, 124:527-534, 1967.

Guteirrez, J.: The gamines of Columbia, In Sixteenth Winter Meeting of the American Academy of Psychoanalysis, New York City, December 3-5, 1971.

Hart, T.: Personal communication.

Heath, D.: Growing Up in College. San Francisco, Jossey-Bass, 1968.

Helson, R.: Sex-specific patterns in creative literary phantasy. J Pers, 38:344-363, 1970.

Herzberg, J.: Urban "family" communes serving youth's moratoria. In Highlights: The 125th Annual Meeting of the American Psychiatric Association, Dallas, Texas, May 1-5, 1972. Psychiatric Spectator, 8: 1972.

Heston, L., and Gottesman, I.: Genetic counseling in psychiatry. Modern Med, May, 1972, pp. 48-52.

Hirsch, S., and Kenniston, K.: Psychosocial issues in talented college dropouts. Psychiatry, 33:1-20, 1970.

Hoffer, W.: Mouth, hand and ego-interaction. In Eissler, R. (Ed.): The Psychoanalytic Study of the Child. New York, Int Univ Pr, 1949, vol. III, pp. 49-56.

Hollan, T.: Poor school performance as symptom of masked depression in children and adolescents. Am J Psychother, 25:258-263, 1970.

Jenkins, R.: Runaway reaction. Am J Psychiatry, 128:168-173, 1971.

Jenkins, R., and Bayer, A.: Types of delinquent behavior and background factors. Int J Soc Psychiatry, 14:65-76, 1968.

Jochmus, I.: Anorexia nervosa in two male adolescents. Prax Kinderpsychol Kinderpsychiatr, 16:1-6, 1967.

Jost, A.: Problems of fetal endocrinology: The gonadal and hypophyseal hormones. Recent Prog Horm Res, 8:379, 1953.

Judd, L., and Maudell, A.: A free clinic population and drug use patterns. Am J Psychiatry, 128:1298-1302, 1972.

Katz, J.: Biological and psychological roots of psychosexual identity. Med Aspects of Human Sexuality, June, 1972, pp 103-110.

Katz, J., et al.: No Time for Youth. San Francisco, Jossey-Bass, 1968.

Kelly, F.: The effectiveness of survival camp training with delinquents. Forty-eighth Annual Meeting, American Orthopsychiatric Association, Washington, D.C., 1971.

Khan, A.: "Mamma's boy" syndrome. Am J Psychiatry, 128:712-717, 1971.

King, S.: Coping mechanisms in adolescents. Psychiatric Annals, 1:10-46, 1971.

Kinsey, A., Pomeroy, W., and Martin, C.: Sexual Behavior in the Human Male. Philadelphia, Saunders, 1948.

Kraus, R.: Emergency evaluation of suicide attempters. Pa Med, April, 1972, pp. 70-72.

Kriesman, D.: Social interaction and intimacy in preschizophrenic adolescence. In Zubin, J., and Freedman, A. (Eds.): The Psychopathology of Adolescence. New York, Grune, 1970.

Larimer, G.: Drugs and youth. Pennsylvania's Health, 32:2-10, Winter, 1971.

Ling, W., et al.: Depressive illness in childhood presenting as severe headache. Am J Dis Child, 120:122-124, 1970.

Lipinski, E.: Motivation in drug misuse: Some comments on agent environment and host. JAMA, 219:171-174, 1972.

Lipp, M., and Benson, S.: Physician use of marijuana, alcohol and tobacco. Am J Psychiatry, 129:612-614, 1972.

Little, R.: Critical issues in the treatment of the physician addict. Philadelphia Med, May, 1972, pp. 339-340.

Louria, D., and Wolfson, E.: Medical complications of drug abuse. Drug Therapy, 2:35-44, 1972.

Maddocks, P.: Five-year follow-up of untreated psychopaths. Br J Psychiatry, 116:511-515, 1970.

Mahler, M.: Thoughts about development and individuation. Psychoanal Study Child, 18:307-324, 1963.

Mannino, F., and Delgado, R.: Trichotillomania in children: a review. Am J Psychiatry, 126:505, 1969.

Marcotte, D.: Marijuana and mutism. Am J Psychiatry, 129:475-476, 1972.

Marijuana clouded their recent memory. In Medical World News, April, 1972.

Masters, W., and Johnson, V.: Human Sexual Response. Boston, Little, 1966.

Masterson, J.: Depression in the adolescent character disorder. In Zubin, J., and Freedman, A. (Eds.): The Psychopathology of Adolescence. New York, Grune, 1970.

Masterson, J.: The Psychiatric Dilemma of Adolescence. Boston, Little, 1967.

McCaffery, T.: Severe growth retardation in children with inflammatory bowel disease. Pediatrics, 45:426-432, 1970.

McDonald, J.: Homicidal threats. Am J Psychiatry, 124:475-482, 1967.

Micks, R.: The essentials of materia medica. In Pharmacology and Therapeutics, 5th ed. London, J and A Churchill Ltd., 1951.

Milstein, F.: Clarifying the patient's sense of identity: Special problems in treating female offenders. Int J Offender Therapy, 15:16-20, 1971.

Money J.: Hormonal and genetic extremes at puberty. In Zubin, J., and Freedman, A. (Eds.): The Psychopathology of Adolescence, New York, Grune, 1970.

Money, J., et al.: An examination of some basic sexual concepts: The evidence of human hermaphroditism. Johns Hopkins Med J, 97:301, 1955.

Murphy, S., and Chapman, W.: Adolescent enuresis: A urological study. Pediatrics, 45:426-432, 1970.

Nadler, R.: Pseudohedonistic syndrome, in "What can be done when the acting-out does not stop?" Bull NY Soc For Adolescent Psychiatry, April, 1972.

Nation, R.: Psychological findings on girls admitted to Cumberlow Lodge. Cumberlow Lodge, London, printed by London Borough of Lambeth, 1968.

Nelson, S.: Follow-up study of wrist-slashers. Am J Psychiatry, 127:1345-1349, 1971.

Newman, L.: Transsexualism in adolescence: problems in evaluation and treatment. Arch Gen Psychiatry, 23:112-121, 1970.

Obese teenager: Family scapegoat. Medical World News, May, 1972, p. 425.

Ottenberg, D.: Modalities of treatment of narcotic addicts. Pa Med, May, 1972, pp. 350-353.

Otto, U.: Suicide among Swedish children and adolescents. In Coplan, G., and Lebovici, S. (Eds.): Adolescence: Psychosocial Perspectives. New York, Basic, 1969.

Palmai, G., et al.: Social class and the young offender. Br J Psychiatry, 113:1073-1082, 1967.

Papavasiliou, P.: Persistent dyskinesias in drug users. JAMA, 271:88-89, 1972.

Penn, A., et al.: Drugs, coma and myoglobinuria. Arch Neurol, 26:336-343, 1972.

Perez-Reyes, M., and Falk, R.: Follow-up of abortion in early adolescents. In Highlights: Twenty-third Annual Meeting of the American Association of Psychiatric Services for Children, Beverly Hills, Calif., Nov. 17-21, 1971.

Pet, D., and Ball, J.: Marijuana smoking in the United States. Federal Probation, 1968.

Reddy, A., et al.: Observations on heroin and methadone withdrawal in newborn. Pediatrics, 43:353-358, 1971.

Redl, F., and Wineman, D.: Children Who Hate. New York, Free Pr, 1951.

Reid, L.: Personal communication.

Rodriguez, et al.: Encephalopathy and paraplegia occurring with use of heroin. New York J Med, 71:2879-2880, 1971.

Rose, G.: Maternal control, superego formation, and identity. In Feinstein, S., Giovacchini, P., and Miller, A. (Eds.): Adolescent Psychiatry. New York, Basic, 1971, vol. I.

Rosenberg, C., and Patch, V.: Methadone use in adolescent heroin addicts. JAMA, 220:991-993, May, 1972.

Rosenthal, R., et al.: Wrist-cutting syndrome: The meaning of a gesture. Am J Psychiatry, 128:1363-1368, 1972.

Rostov, M.: Death by suicide in hospital: Analysis of twenty therapeutic failures. Am J Psychother, 25:216-227, 1970.

Rovinsky, J.: Abortion in New York City: Preliminary experience with permissive abortion statute. Obstet Gynecol, 38:333-342, 1971.

Runaway children. In U.S. News and World Report. New York, April, 1972, pp. 38-42.

Russell, D.: On the psychopathology of boy prostitutes. Int J Offender Therapy, 15:49-52, 1971.

Salzman, L.: Changing styles in psychiatric syndromes. In Highlights: 125th Annual Meeting of the American Psychiatric Association, Dallas, Texas, May 1-5, 1972. Psychiatric Spectator, 7:11-14.

Sanborn, D.: Drug abusers, suicide attempters and the MMPI. Dis Nerv Syst, 32:183-187, 1971.

Sanderson, G., and Hall-Smith, P.: Tonsure trichotillomania. Br J Dermatol, 82:343-350, 1970.

Schmideberg, M.: Personal communication.

Schmideberg, M.: Promiscuous and rootless girls. Int J Offender Therapy, 15:28-33, 1971.

Selzer, M., et al.: Fatal accidents: Role of psychopathology, social stress and acute disturbance. Am J Psychiatry, 124:1028-1036, 1968.

Senay, E.: Therapeutic abortion: Clinical aspects. Arch Gen Psychiatry, 23:408-415, 1970.

Shainess, N.: Toward a new feminine psychology. CMD, April, 1972, pp. 393-402.

Shapiro, A.: Gilles de la tourette's disease. Am J Psychiatry, 129:99, 1972.

Shapiro, R.: Adolescent ego autonomy and the family. In Caplan, G., and Lebovici, S. (Eds.): Adolescence: Psychosocial Perspectives. New York, Basic, 1969.

Shearn, C., and Fitzgibbons, D.: Patterns of drug use in a population of youthful psychiatric patients. Am J Psychiatry, 128:1381-1387, 1972.

Sherman, J.: What men do not know about women's sexuality. Med Aspects of Human Sexuality, November, 1972.

Shore, J., et al.: A suicide prevention center on an Indian reservation. Am J Psychiatry, 128:76-81, 1972.

Silver, M.: Relation of depression to attempted suicide and seriousness of intent. Arch Gen Psychiatry, 25:573-576, 1971.

Sklansky, M., et al.: The High School Adolescent. New York, Assn Pr, 1969.

Slawson, P., and Davidson, P. III: Hysterical self-mutilation of the tongue. Arch Gen Psychiatry, 11:581-589, 1964.

Smith, S.: The adolescent murdered. Arch Gen Psychiatry, 13:310-319, 1965.

Stoak, M.: Antisocial juveniles from orderly families. Dtsch Z Ges Gericht Med, 62:108-113, 1968.

Stoller, R.: The term "transvestism." Arch Gen Psychiatry, 24:230-237, 1971.

Szasz, T.: Psychoanalysis and the autonomic nervous system. Psychoanal Rev, 39:115, 1952.

Talbott, J., and Teague, J.: Marijuana psychosis. JAMA, 210:299-302, 1969.

Thibault, A.: The group and the adolescent: its usual significance and its contemporary evolution. Laral Med, 39:118-126, 1968.

Thrasher, F., and Short, J.: The Gang. Chicago, Chicago University Press, 1962.

Tolpin, P.: Some psychic determinants of orgiastic dysfunction. In Feinstein, S., Giovacchini, P., and Miller, A. (Eds.): Adolescent Psychiatry. New York, Basic, 1971.

Toolan, J.: Depression in children and adolescents. In Caplan, G., and Lebovici, S. (Eds.): Adolescence: Psychosocial Perspectives. New York, Basic, 1969.

Toolan, J.: Changes in the personality structure during adolescence. In Masserman, J. (Ed.): Science and Psychoanalysis. New York, Grune, 1960, vol. III.

Ulmar, G.: Adolescent girls who steal. Rev Neuropsychiatr Infant, 18:439-459, 1970.

Vaillant, G.: What kinds of men get psychosomatic illness? In Highlights: Annual Meeting of the American Psychosomatic Society, Boston, Mass., April 14-16, 1972. Psychiatric Spectator, 8:17-18.

Vandervort, W., and Paulshock, B.: Laboratory screening of heroin addicts. JAMA, 220:1014, 1972.

Vidal, G., and Smulerer, D.: Childhood bereavement and mental disorders. Acta Psyquat Amer Lat, 16:62-66, 1970.

Wardrop, K.: Delinquent teenage types. Brit J Criminol, 7:371-380, 1967.

Wenzel, R.: Venn diagrams in drug abuse education. JAMA, 220:860-861, 1972.

Westlake, W., and Epstein, N.: The Silent Majority. San Francisco, Jossey-Bass, 1968.

Whitehead, C.: Pseudowithdrawal observed among methadone patients. Psychiat News, April, 1972.

Whitney, W.: Depressive symptoms and academic performance in college students. Am J Psychiat, 128:748-760, December 1971.

Wiener, J.: The regrets of children. Psychiat Annals, 2:12-18, September, 1972.

Wikler, A.: Opiod addiction. In Freedman, A., and Kaplan, H. (Eds.): Comprehensive Textbook of Psychiatry. Baltimore, Williams & Wilkins, 1967

Wilson, M.: A proposed diagnostic classification for adolescent psychiatric cases. In Feinstein, S., Giovacchini, P., and Miller, A. (Eds.): Adolescent Psychiatry. New York, Basic, 1971, vol. I, pp. 275-295.

Wilschke, K.: Biting as an early symptom of aggressiveness in juvenile delinquents. Dtsch Z Ges Gerichtl Med, 62:116-119, 1968.

Zallemore, J., and Wilson, W.: Adolescent maladjustment or affective disorder. Am J Psychiat, 129:608-612, November, 1972.

CHAPTER IV

TREATMENT OF THE ADOLESCENT

Definition

TREATMENT of the adolescent constitutes the use of one or a combination of therapeutic interventions to relieve stress, alleviate symptoms and foster resumption of psychological development and adaptational pursuits.

PRESENTING PROBLEMS

The following classification is empirical and reflects some of the more common bases for seeking clinical help for the adolescent.

A. *Acute*
1. Self-destructiveness: Suicide attempt, psychogenic accidents.
2. Violence: Assault with or without a weapon; with or without psychosis.
3. Panic: Hetero- or homosexual.
4. Legal Crisis: Court-ordered period of psychiatric evaluation.
5. Drug Crisis: Overdose, withdrawal or psychosis.
6. School Crisis: Suspension, failure or expulsion.
7. Family Crisis: Breakup, violence, death, incest, pregnancy, runaway.
8. Psychotic Crisis: Acute depression or schizophrenia.

B. *Subacute*
1. Psychosis: Depressive, schizophrenic.
2. Neurosis: Severe anxiety, obsessionalism or compulsivity.
3. Withdrawal Behavior: From family, friends; with/ without drug use.
4. "Unhappiness:" Usually reflecting crisis of values, low self-esteem and a failure orientation; related to problems

of dependency, identification, deprivation and depression.

5. Drug Addiction: With impairment of function and social relations.

6. Minor delinquency: Disturbance to the family or community with minor offenses and less than two arrests.

C. *Chronic*

1. Retardation with related adaptational difficulties.
2. Organic brain syndrome — often drug related.
3. Epilepsy-related adaptational difficulties.
4. Psychosis with regressive or bizarre behavior.

ASSESSMENT OF MOTIVATION

The Precontract Negotiation

The mere presentation of the young patient to the clinician does not always imply his readiness to become involved with and committed to protracted psychotherapy. Nor does it suggest his acceptance of the concept that he has a psychological problem.

If Winnicott (1960) and Evans (personal communication) refer to the "treatment contract" or concretization of a working therapeutic relationship between the therapist, the adolescent and the interested third party, the "precontract negotiation" assesses the motivation for the referral.

Initial contact between the clinician and the young person may represent the adolescent's own initiative, the initiative of his family of that of another party. The source of the impetus and the motivation behind it are important issues to clarify for the clinician right from the outset. It helps him to determine if treatment can proceed and succeed.

Adolescent-Initiated Contact

The young person may seek out the psychotherapist or counselor himself. This is occurring more frequently on the college campus, in military service, and at community health facilities.

Basic motivations for such self-referrals are psychological pain and/or an increasing dissatisfaction with status quo. On the other hand, the clinician must be aware of the patient's possible manipulativeness and the quest for secondary gain via therapeutic contact. This usually occurs in the face of an impending crisis where credit for seeking psychological help would favorably influence the outcome, e.g. a judge will often waive sentencing someone arrested for drug use if the adolescent seeks psychiatric help. During the Vietnamese War, some young men had sought psychological help as a means of demonstrating their unsuitability for military service. Heroin addicts may request hospitalization simply to detoxify and reduce the size of their habit rather than to break their addiction. Thus, the therapist must consider the young person's request for help not only in terms of need but also in terms of motivation.

Family-Initiated Contact

Here again assessment of the motivation of the interceding family member is of paramount importance not only in determining the feasibility of treating the adolescent in question but also in formulating a valid treatment approach. The family call may reflect genuine concern, but it may also signify rejection of or anger toward the young patient; and the therapist's task under such conditions is most difficult.

The family call may reflect more: It may be a covert call for help for the whole family masked by focus on the adolescent, the family's "official" patient. Involvement of significant family members requires much tact and patience. Selling the concept that the adolescent's crisis may reflect family problems is crucial in such cases.

Institution-Initiated Contact

The greater the feeling of coercion or humiliation on the part of the adolescent "sent" for treatment, the less likelihood there is that he will ever lend himself to a therapeutic endeavor. Thus, institutional motivation for the referral is important and the young person's perception of the event must not be ignored.

The teacher, the employer, or the court may send the adolescent to a psychotherapeutic facility out of compassion and concern. Such referrals may also be made out of the desire to be rid of a headache, and the chances for meaningful psychotherapy under these negative circumstances are questionable. This is illustrated time and again when the courts remand juvenile offenders to psychiatric hospitals by default because more appropriate facilities are not available. Evans (personal communication) and Schmideberg (personal communication) both report on the therapeutic ineffectiveness of such dispositions.

In general then, where the motivation for referral of the young patient to the psychotherapist or treatment facility is ambivalent or negative, effective psychological treatment is difficult. While the therapist might readily acknowledge a need for care in such situations, all he may be able to accomplish is to define the psychological problem, the motivational complications, and the difficulties in the therapeutic task. At times, postponement of treatment until a more conducive time is a valid tactic.

THE SPECIAL NATURE OF ADOLESCENT TREATMENT

Treatment of the emotionally disturbed adolescent is unique in many ways. The following table compares adolescent psychotherapy with that of the child and the adult.

Psychological treatment of the adolescent presents a unique situation (Schoenfeld, 1970). His circumstances are special, as he is usually beholden to someone else for support, although acknowledgement of his multiple dependencies is highly conflictual and the cause of much difficulty in therapy (Welsch, 1957).

The psychology of the adolescent and his special needs are different from both those of the child and the adult, and special therapeutic techniques are required to cope with these needs, those of the family and with the demands of external reality. Management of drug problems, manipulativeness, the propensity to act out, school pressures, family crises, and the requirements of the society render psychological treatment of young people a highly unique subspecialty.

Table I: Special Nature of Adolescent Treatment

Parameter of Treatment	Adult	Adolescent	Child
Legal	Responsible	*Dependent	Dependent
Financial	Responsible	*Dependent	Dependent
Life Pattern	Stable	Transitional	Stable
Family Involvement	Secondary	*Primary	Primary
Referral Source	Usually Self	Rarely Self	Never Self
Psychotherapeutic Technique	1) Supportive or Reconstructive	1) Usually Supportive	1) Usually Supportive
	2) Orthodox, adult techniques and standard language	2) Variable unorthodox techniques with special adolescent idiom	2) Orthodox play format with simple standard language
Role of Medications	Often Important	Variable	Occasionally Important
Duration of Treatment	Often full course	Often interrupted	Often full course
Drug Addiction as Complicating Factor	Unusual	Often	Unusual
Acting out as a complicating factor	Unusual	Often	Unusual
Goals	Removal of Pathology	Resumption of Development	Resumption of Development

*Except when emancipated

Goals of Adolescent Treatment

The adolescent patient is in a transitional phase of life psychologically, physiologically and socially, and the objectives of therapy reflect this state of flux. Schoenfeld (1970) writes of the need to alter symptoms as a goal of therapy, and Beres (1964) notes their shifting, transitory nature.

Wolf (1970), Sklansky (1969) and Robbins (1960) focus on the need to help the adolescent solve current reality problems and foster ego growth as well as cope with problems of conscience.

Erikson (1968) notes the importance of resolving problems of identity, and Berman (1957) cites the need to help improve adolescent-parent relationships and aid in planning for the future.

Josselyn (1957) points out, and many authors concur, that deep insight is often not necessary and often too upsetting for the young patient to cope with. Holmes (1969) elaborates the importance of limit setting for the acting out adolescent, and Rinsley (1971) stresses the need to manage resistances as well as educate the young person about his psychological problem. Each clinician conceptualizes the essence and goal of treatment in his own way. In general, these objectives may be summarized as follows:

A. Provide relief from stressful feelings, symptoms or behavior.
B. Foster resumption of ego development:
    1. In the area of education and preparation of a life's work.
    2. In the area of gender identity formation and the ability to form meaningful, long-term heterosexual relationships.
    3. In the area of social skills and the ability to form friendly, give-and-take relationships.
C. Improve function and coping techniques and solve personal problems.
D. Avoid psychological material that would overwhelm defenses and produce panic.

The following therapeutic vignette is illustrative of complications resulting from the sudden unleashing of deep unconscious material.

Case

Arthur was a twenty-year-old dilettante college student who was referred to the psychiatrist for his general unhappiness and underachievement. Initial evaluation revealed a young man who was almost symbiotically dependent upon his equally dependent mother; Arthur's father seemed both angry and distant.

Arthur's college dysfunction seemed to be a reflection of his inner expectation that things would be done for him by someone else, somehow. His problems of dependency produced not only submarginal college performance but also failure to win girlfriends. So long as the therapeutic focus was upon girls and scholarship, the positive therapeutic relationship and some insights helped him attack the problem of dependency productively. The therapeutic course changed dramatically when the patient brought in a series of dreams dealing with erotic feelings about mother and about men. Their Oedipal and homosexual implications were obvious to Arthur. Instead of veering away from this material and refocusing upon girls and grades, the therapist pursued a deeper insight. Anxiety mounted dramatically and sessions were missed for the first time. Arthur soon announced that inasmuch as exams were forthcoming, he was stopping treatment, as he wanted to devote all his time to his work. A more tangential and delicate treatment of the unconscious instinctual material would have forestalled the panic and interruption of treatment.

BASIC CONCEPTS OF ADOLESCENT TREATMENT

A. *Psychodynamic frame of reference* — This implies a comprehension of human development and psychological behavior derived from the psychoanalytic literature. It is predicated upon the importance of childhood experiences; parental relationships; behavior that is, in part, derived from unconscious drives and conflicts; and the transitional nature of adolescent biology and psychology (Welsch, 1957; Searles, 1960).

B. *Therapeutic techniques that are flexible and variable* — Orthodoxy and rigidity of technique are usually unrewarded as each adolescent patient requires his own special approach.

C. *Therapeutic objectives of ego-strengthening and resumption of ego development.* (Wolf, 1970; Sklansky, 1969; Robbins, 1960).

D. *Special stance for the therapist* — The style of treatment that the therapist employs is of critical importance. The following qualities are considered desirable: An open, direct, informal approach, a helpful giving manner, an active orientation that allows variation and thwarts boredom, as well as the projection of an image of easy accessibility that fosters identification by the young person. (Searles, 1960; Samorajczyk, 1971). (See page 108)

E. *Continuum of care facilities* — Care for the young person often requires a variety of physical settings and facilities to properly deal with his needs.

Hospitalization in a special residential setting is often indicated to remove the adolescent from a noxious situation and permit the forces of treatment to be mustered. Remedial education and vocational training are essential parameters of adolescent care. An alternative domicile that is semi-structured and sheltered is frequently necessary after hospital discharge (Caplan, 1969).

F. *Family involvement* — Treatment of the adolescent requires evaluation of the primary family unit, not only to enlist its support, but also to determine what role it has played in contributing to the young person's pathology.

The degree to which each family should become involved in the overall treatment regimen varies according to each particular situation. Minimum family involvement is indicated when the adolescent is older and/or strongly opposed to their involvement. When the adolescent is younger and more dependent and there is obvious and strong psychopathology among family members, their inclusion in a treatment plan is warranted. Formulae for involvement too, are variable. When the therapist is sufficiently experienced, he may treat all of the family members at different times and to different degrees. If it is decided that other therapists are to be involved, constant communication between therapists is vital to minimize the tendency to polarize and manipulate on the part of different family members.

The one-time popular view that the family of the adolescent was to be cordoned off from the field of treatment and rendered innocuous no longer seems tenable. Judicious family involvement is often an important element of therapeutic success.

Settings

From an evolutional point of view, treatment camps for

delinquents and child guidance centers are amongst the earliest facilities developed for the care of disturbed adolescents (Aichorn, 1953; Makareno, 1936; Kelly, 1971).

Educational institutions now offer increasing psychological help. Sklansky (1969) and Peltz (1957), among others, describe diagnostic and therapeutic efforts at the level of secondary education. Kenniston (1971), Farnsworth, Arnstein (1971), etc. describe treatment on the college campus. Rinsley (1971), Balser (1957) and Hendrickson, et al. (1959) deal with treatment in a residential hospital setting, and Holmes (1969), Josselyn (1957), Blos (1970), and many others, report on psychotherapy of the young person on an outpatient basis.

Treatment facilities for young people may be categorized as follows:

A. *Community Facilities*
   1. *Outpatient*
      a. Private care.
      b. General hospital outpatient clinics.
      c. Community mental health center clinics.
      d. Voluntary community agencies for crisis intervention, e.g. HELP.
      e. Veterans Administration Hospital clinics.
   2. *Transitional* (offering partial hospitalization)
      a. Private hostels (shelters) e.g. The Rebecca Gratz Home for Women in Philadelphia.
      b. Church run hostels, e.g. Sisters of the Good Shepherd.
      c. Community mental health center day care programs.
B. *Hospital Facilities* (Inpatient)
   1. Private psychiatric hospitals with or without a special adolescent unit or program.
   2. State mental hospital with or without a special adolescent unit or program.
   3. General hospital psychiatric wing, usually without special facilities for young patients.
   4. Veterans administration hospital psychiatric wing.
   5. Special state psychiatric facility for children and adolescents e.g., Eastern State School and Hospital, Ben Salem Township, PA.

C. *Educational Facilities*
  1. Secondary School Level:
     a. Diagnostic and counseling services.
     b. Special classes for emotionally disturbed students.
     c. Special schools for emotionally disturbed youth, e.g. Devereux Foundation.
  2. College Level:
     a. College psychiatric service.
     b. College counseling service.
D. *Military Facilities*
E. *Facilities in Business Enterprises*
  1. Diagnostic and evaluative service.
  2. Encounter groups.
F. *Correctional Facilities or Units*
  1. Short term detention centers with access to diagnostic and treatment facilities.
  2. Juvenile correctional institutions with treatment facilities, often insufficient.
G. *Specialized Facilities* e.g. for mental retardates, etc.

FORMS OF PSYCHOLOGICAL TREATMENT

The field of adolescent care is relatively new, yet the therapeutic armamentarium is already considerable. But if many types of treatment are available, more research needs to be done to refine them further and to establish clear-cut indications and contraindications for their use.

The Special Role of the Hospital

In the final analysis, the objective of a therapeutic intervention is to effect change that is both lasting and constructive. Sometimes the cumulative impact of several forms of treatment are necessary before emotional growth and development can occur, especially with young people seriously involved with drugs or manifesting major behavior disorders. In such situations, treatment in a residential hospital setting is advisable. Other indications for hospitalization are the need to remove the young person from a noxious environmental situation, to clinically observe an adolescent who might pose a diagnostic problem, or to marshall family support via the dramatic gesture of hospitalization. It is this author's impression that care of the disturbed young patient is often facilitated in a proper residential setting which offers all the outpatient treatment modalities as well as many important forms of therapy only available in an intramural setting.

The following list of treatment forms are by no means mutually exclusive. Frequently, the greatest therapeutic success is achieved by the simultaneous use of several forms of treatment. Of the following therapies, all can be practiced in an inpatient, outpatient or partial hospitalization setting, although milieu therapy and the allied therapies are usually reserved for the hospital.

One-to-One Psychotherapy

This form of psychological treatment can be the most profound and conducive of insight and personality change. It lends itself to the formation of strong transference relationships and corrective identifications. It is usually based on the psychodynamic or psychoanalytic model which requires special training in adolescent care. Other forms of one-to-one psychotherapy are employed and render the valuable services of ego support, guidance, symptom control and reality-oriented problem solving.

With a well-motivated patient, psychotherapy can be an effective tool in treating adolescent neuroses and psychoses, especially since psychopathology is less fixed and more labile in the adolescent. However, with major delinquents (more than two arrests) and major drug users (prolonged use, biological stigmata, and the denial of psychological problems), motivation is often poor and psychotherapy, as the sole therapeutic tool, is less effective.

Group Psychotherapy

Peer grouping is a natural phenomenon of the adolescent phase and the formation of such cliques for therapeutic purposes can be very effective (Berkovitz, 1972). Once adolescents develop a group spirit, treatment can pursue a variety of forms and objectives.

McWhinnie (1969) delineates five phases of adolescent group therapy in his work with institutionalized delinquents: (1) Catharsis or the revelation of one's own story, (2) testing of staff regarding confidentiality and their capacity to set and maintain limits, (3) group identity formation, (4) resistance, (5) the definition of personal problems. Elaboration of these phases, however, is predicated upon relatively prolonged stays in a closed residential setting and may not otherwise be apparent.

The clustering of young people together into a psychological union may produce a powerful social force with much positive potential for emotional growth and development. This same social group, however, may also develop regressive and destructive tendencies (Caplan, 1969; Wolf, 1970). Thus, it is imperative for the therapist to be alert to the possibility of antisocial group formation and acting out (destructive behavior that is conscious or unconscious, often repetitive and reflective of conflict).

To foster therapeusis and thwart destructive behavior, the following maneuvers may be helpful:

1. *Control the overall milieu:* This can best be achieved in a closed setting operating within the context of a milieu, the values of which support and reinforce the positive endeavors of the group.

2. *Provide group leaders of sufficient skill and numbers:* Teichers (1966), Fenton (1957) and others all cite the need for experience and skill on the part of the leader. At times, sufficient numbers of co-therapists are necessary to keep the group moving in the right direction, especially when the number of young patients exceeds eight and several of them have shown antisocial tendencies.

3. *Provide balance and variety to groups:* It may be helpful at times to disperse antisocial cliques among other therapeutic groups to discourage acting out. It may also be helpful to expose adolescents to mixed chronological groups to broaden their experience and discourage regressive behavior.

General indications for group psychotherapy are the need for positive group identification, the development of social skills, and the definition of personal problems. Where sufficient time is available, solutions to the defined problems can be attempted under the supervision and guidance of the group leaders.

Contraindications for group psychotherapy are few: disruptiveness of the group by virtue of psychosis and/or antisocial behavior and exploitation of fellow patients by psychopathic patients.

Milieu Therapy

Milieu therapy is a form of treatment derived from exposure to a special environment which espouses and promulgates values productive of mental health and positive social interaction. It may operate in a variety of settings such as special camps, day care centers, and hospitals and is more effective in a closed environment where values and rules can be enforced.

Historically, milieu therapy derived its inspiration from Maxwell Jones' pioneering efforts in the therapeutic community at the Dingleton Hospital in Scotland. Basic concepts of Jones' program consisted of an active treatment program, the patient playing an important role in his treatment, and the development of interdisciplinary teams (Jones, 1962). Further refinements in milieu therapy were developed at the Sheppard and Enoch Pratt Hospital where the psychiatrist's role was split and divided into administrative and therapeutic functions (Stanton, 1960). This dichotomy allowed the treating physician to dissociate himself from dealing with problems of authority, thereby facilitating his therapeutic efforts.

For the adolescent inpatient, milieu therapy is an important aspect of a total therapeutic hospital experience, as it provides him with valuable guidelines for social interaction as well as a set of viable and useful values to live by.

In defining the therapeutic milieu, Jones (1962) and Auerswald (1969) stress the need to view the institution in its entirety in assessing the impact upon the patient. Cumming and Cumming (1962) elaborate this point further by citing the importance of a well-defined social structure and participation both by staff and patients in the therapeutic program in order to insure successful interaction. Gralnick (1962) cites the need to include family therapy and the multidisciplinary team as basic elements of milieu therapy. Berman (1957) adds education, psychotherapy and social development to the above and Greaves and Regan (1957) stress the value of a full day's activities as part of a therapeutic milieu for hospitalized young people.

Other facets of milieu therapy hinge upon reality testing (Robinson, Vanderpol, 1960), the establishment of a sense of belonging (Washburn, 1960), and even upon structural design which should produce a sense of belonging and familiarity amongst the patients. (Novick, 1971).

The milieu, however, must cater specifically to the needs of the particular patient population. Thus, the design of the milieu must change to meet changing patient needs (Jorsted, personal communication).

Problems may develop in the therapeutic milieu due to a declining morale of the staff; this can occur when the chain of command and responsibilities are blurred, when authority and roles change (Rubenstein, 1971), or when polarization of the staff into competitive segments occurs (Searles, 1960). In fact, any stress impacting upon any part of the hospital community which functions as a closed system, will be reflected often in negative staff feelings, producing a profound influence upon the climate of the hospital and the emotional tone of the patients. This has been demonstrated again and again in terms of the content of inpatient group therapy sessions during periods of hospital stress or dissension.

Milieu Therapy: Résumé

1. Milieu therapy is a highly important mode of treatment for the adolescent in terms of his need for more adaptive values and objects to identify with.

2. It functions better in a closed (hospital) community that is internally consistent regarding the implicit and explicit values it espouses.

3. Four major areas of activity of the milieu are therapeutic, educational, social and personal.

4. A well-coordinated, multidisciplinary staff, operating in a harmonious setting is essential, and a conducive warm interior

design no doubt plays a significant role.

5. The therapeutic milieu must be flexible and adapt to the special needs of its patient population.

6. A full day of meaningful activity is essential for a hospitalized adolescent and an important part of the therapeutic milieu.

7. The therapeutic climate for patients may be upset by stresses interposed at any point in the closed social system of the hospital community.

Family Therapy

Indications for extending psychological treatment to a family unit rather than restricting it to an individual patient has been elucidated by Ackerman and Behrens (1958), Bowen and other pioneers of the field. Caplan (1969) and Kaplan (1969) see the family approach as an essential means of insuring support for work with the primary patient, clarifying his diagnosis, facilitating communication among all concerned parties, and decreasing family guilt. Ackerman and Behrens (1958) and Harms (1965) can only understand individual behavior in the context of family process, and Berman (1957) and Auerswald (1969) find family therapy a necessary part of adolescent care.

Lewis (1971) describes the healthy family as one where:

1. Family leadership is in the hands of both parents interacting cooperatively and positively.

2. Communication is clear.

3. Emotional warmth is more important than hostility.

4. Problem-solving thinking predominates.

5. Achievement of individual autonomy is a family value.

The need to understand individual behavior as a function of family dynamics is illustrated in the following vignette.

Case

Stuart, a sixteen-year-old urbanite, was remanded by the court to a mental hospital for having slashed another school boy with a piece of broken glass in a maniacal rage. During the course of the hospitalization, he experienced auditory hallucinations for the first time and manifested bizarre behavior as well as the capacity to get other patients to physically beat him. In psychotherapy, he provided much material dealing with identificational confusion and had been involved in a number of overt homosexual experiences since puberty.

Family evaluation revealed a father with striking problems of passive dependency, a history of episodes of violent rage in which Stuart was beaten sadistically, as well as the dynamics of a homosexual problem that was partly conscious.

Stuart's mother was chronically depressed and had withdrawn sullenly and resignedly many years before. In the process, she also withdrew from Stuart who perceived this as abandonment.

Despite the major psychopathology evident in the family, all wanted treatment of some form, although both parents initially needed to believe that their involvement was to facilitate their son's therapy.

With this particular primary group, the formula for family treatment consisted of initial focus upon Stuart, the "identified" patient, and gradually increasing inclusion of the parents. The father-son dyad received particular attention to allow Stuart to express his rage non-masochistically for the first time. Part of Stuart's therapeutic task consisted of differentiating psychotic thinking from secondary process mental activity. In addition, he reduced his titer of anxiety via support from his psychiatrist as well as the reduction of the threat from father. Identification with the male therapist diminished the attractiveness of the homosexual solution to his sex drive and he began to develop active interests in women, first for a mother figure and later for a heterosexual partner.

Stuart's father enjoyed the peer relationship with encouragement from the doctor-authority figure and felt secure enough to confront his own problems of sadism, passivity and male identification. As he began to feel stronger in his masculinity, he was able to become more giving and paternal to Stuart.

Stuart's mother also derived support from the therapeutic relationship and shifted from the position of the stifled depressive to the angry wife capable of overt expression of feeling. Treatment of this family unit is ongoing at this writing. Without involvement of both parents, Stuart's progress would have been considerably hampered if not impossible.

Brown's family therapy (1970) focuses upon reality problems, family dynamics and the need to reduce resistances, guilt and anxiety. This same approach proved most effective with Stuart's family.

Many theoretical approaches to family therapy exist. Haley categorizes them as (1) analytic, with focus on the one to one therapeutic relationship; (2) the systems approach which eschews individual psychodynamics and deals with group process; and (3) an intermediate approach which combines features of both.

Modified techniques to meet different situations will continue to evolve. Family therapy in a residential treatment setting must take cognizance of such factors as hospital stays that are frequently brief, family units that are often fragmented or partially available, and a relatively large number of young patients to be served. Yet, a family approach that includes treating several adolescents, and their families for brief periods of time has been shown to be effective and could become an important aspect of the adolescent care. This "multiple family-fragment therapy" often helps by establishing communication among family members, clarifying key issues, and precipitating confrontations under controlled conditions. Covert problems become openly defined and thus constitutes the first step towards resolution.

Family patterns of interaction may change and pathological relationships may be broken as a consequence with a resultant improvement in the adolescent primary patient.

Adjunctive Therapy

The field of adjunctive therapy is of inestimable value in the treatment of the adolescent, yet its importance has often gone without proper acknowledgement (Winn, personal communication; Stern, personal communication). In the context of modern residential treatment, which places so high a premium on the importance of self-expression and the therapeutic team, the adjunctive therapies are playing a more important role.

Several factors contribute to adjunctive therapy's apparently insufficient recognition:

1. *Heterogeniety:* Many disparate disciplines are subsumed under the heading "adjunctive therapy" suggesting a cohesiveness that is more illusory than real. Its very multiplicity of names illustrates the vagueness of the concept, e.g. adjunctive therapy, allied therapy and social therapy. Adjunctive therapists can be specialists in art, music, dance, and recreational and occupational skills; and all of these functions aid the patient in his ability to express himself, to function better, and ultimately to heal himself.

2. *Absence of a professional literature:* The field of psychiatry as well as other areas of the mental health field is often underexposed to adjunctive therapy and is often insufficiently aware of what it can accomplish. As a consequence, the latter is not fully appreciated or utilized.

The functions of adjunctive therapy in an adolescent treatment center are several:

1. *Non-verbal expression:* The spoken word is but one form of expression. It frequently fails as a mode of communication between the therapist and the adolescent patient for many reasons. Thus, the importance of the different forms of non-verbal expression becomes clear. Expression through the different media of adjunctive therapy such as art, music, dance and occupational tasks plays a great role in involving the young patient in his new milieu, in helping him to communicate with others and in effecting a salutary catharsis of emotions that had been long pent up.

2. *Diagnosis and therapeusis:* Styles of function and artistic expression often reflect the patient's psychopathology. In the hands of a skilled and specially trained adjunctive therapist, the special problems of the patient can be illustrated to him via his various productions.

In those treatment centers fostering the therapeutic team concept, the adjunctive therapist's input is often of great value.

3. *Forms of patient expression:* The patient's productions in adjunctive therapy may be categorized in two ways:

EXPRESSIVE — where the particular form of adjunctive therapy produces a true representation of the patient's feelings and psychological dynamics.

RESISTIVE — where the production is either absent or

stereotyped and is not reflective of true expression. It indicates a defensive-resistive posture.

From a longitudinal standpoint, the patient's expressive productions may serve as a sensitive bell-weather of dynamic shifts and changes in the patient occurring during the course of treatment.

In résumé, the adjunctive therapies represent an important segment of the total therapeutic experience. They foster involvement, communication and expression; can aid in diagnosis; and can function as a non-verbal modality for therapeusis.

THE ROLE OF MEDICATIONS

The effectiveness of medication in the treatment of emotionally disturbed adolescents is a function of chemical properties, physiological responses, psychological factors, and the bias of individual reporters (Kraft, 1968). Clinicians committed to psychodynamic and environmental approaches place little importance upon chemical agents and may omit mention of them completely in describing their treatment approach (French, 1963; Mulvaney, 1970). Other clinicians are quite enthusiastic about their results with drugs in treating psychological disorders of adolescence (Fish, 1968; Polack and Laycob, 1971; Rinsley, 1971).

Types of Drugs

Three major classes of drugs used in adolescent psychiatry are tranquilizers, antidepressants and counter-toxic agents. While indications and dosage are generally the same for both young people and adults, relatively little literature is available dealing with the pharmacology of adolescence per se (Reidenberg, personal communication), and drug effects may indeed be different (Taylor and Levine, 1971; O'Malley, et al., 1971).

Psychological Factors

The adolescent's attitude towards the physician and his

medications often plays an important role in drug effectiveness. Katz (1970) points out that young people often view medicine prescribed by the doctor as a symbol of adult authority and reject it. ". . . adolescents tend to resent domination by adults and many see tranquilizers as a means whereby the adult world is attempting to control them." Neff (1971) notes that powerful medications may alter the patient's alertness and sense of reality, thereby evoking further anxiety and even psychosis. The young patient then frequently views the doctor's prescriptions in a special way and his expectations and preconceptions profoundly influence the drug effect. Bergman (1971) illustrates how psychological and sociological factors effect a pharmacological agent; he cites the low incidence of emotional disturbance and adverse side effects among peyote-using Navajo Indians. Use of this drug is socially supported and not an outlawed practice, thereby providing much psychological buttressing to its users and producing fewer adverse side effects.

In general, then, prescriptions of medications to emotionally disturbed young people often produces uneven results, and this is believed attributable to psychological as well as physiological factors. The expectations of the clinician or researcher are also important.

Tranquilizers

While the literature on major and minor tranquilizers is vast, only recently have there been articles devoted to this group of medications and their effect upon the adolescent patient per se. Fish (1968) and Polak and Laycob (1971) note the value of phenothiazines in cases of extreme anxiety. Blumenthal (1971) finds them important in the treatment of gross behavioral disturbances, and Koblenzer (1969) and others report success with phenothiazines in treating young patients with acute schizophrenoid disturbances.

Dosage should be individualized, taking into account the patient's age, weight and intensity of symptoms. The initial trial dose, then, can be altered to suit the needs of the patient.

The use of intramuscular phenothiazines for extreme agitation or assaultiveness, as with the adult, is highly effective. Hypotension is a side effect to be considered and observation of the blood pressure before and after the injection is a wise precaution.

Diphenylhydramine (Benadryl®), chlordiazepoxide (Librium®) and Diazepam (Valium®) have been helpful in the less severe anxiety states (Fish, 1968). Here, too, dosage should be titrated in terms of the individual patient, his symptoms and the desired end result.

Antidepressants

Ling cites the effectiveness of amitriptyline (Elavil®) and imipramine (Tofranil®) in the control of adolescent depression, and this author has found methylphenidate (Ritalin®) of help.

Inasmuch as adolescent depressiveness is a labile symptom, the clinician should be on his guard for a sudden shift to tenseness and anxiety and the need to alter dosages and/or medications appropriately.

Drug Abuse Medications

These are a heterogeneous group of medications used to combat the addictive or toxic effects of drugs taken by young people.

Methadone is a synthetic drug used as a substitute for the opiates. Its advantage is that it provides the addict with longer periods of productivity than the opiates do. The disadvantage is, however, that it is also an addictive drug. When used for purposes of maintenance, it creates an iatrogenic addiction, albeit one that is more manageable. Many clinicians are opposed to this treatment approach for the adolescent addict.

Methadone is also used to detoxify addicts via tapering dosage to a point where the patient is drug free.

The use of methadone, itself an addicting drug, has produced illegal trafficking and problems of abuse and its use has become subject, appropriately, to rather stringent controls. Many investigators have found that the treatment of drug addicts by pharmacological methods alone is unsatisfactory (Fitzpatrick, 1972; Dole, 1972; Gould, 1971); this is especially true for the adolescent and young adult.

Two other families of drugs used in opiate addiction are those that chemically block opiate action and those that antagonize their action. Both of these groups are in the experimental phase, however.

Periods of acute distress resulting from the ingestion of lysergic acid (LSD) are relieved by phenothiazines, and Muller (1971) reports the successful treatment of LSD psychosis with thioridazine.

Acute anxiety and paranoid ideation resulting from amphetamines can be controlled with barbiturates and chloral hydrate (Greenspoon and Hedblom, 1971).

Barbiturate addiction may be treated with gradual withdrawal over ten to fourteen days and overdose, which depresses the vital centers and is potentially life-endangering, often requires hospitalization.

In résumé, then, medications play a significant role in the treatment of emotionally disturbed adolescents. Their importance varies with the kind of problem and with the individual patient.

Young people often discount the importance of or distrust the drugs offered by the adult psychiatrist.

Medications have a definite place in the treatment of severe emotional disorders and acute, drug-induced disorders.

Treatment of drug addiction by drugs alone is usually inadequate and probably will require the use of other modalities as well.

The psychotherapies are of major significance in the restoration of the adolescent to normal psychological development.

BIBLIOGRAPHY

Ackerman, N., and Behrens, M.: The family group and family therapy. In Masserman, J., and Moreno, J. (Eds.): Progress in Psychotherapy. New York, Grune, 1958, vol. 3.

Aichorn, A.: Wayward Youth. New York, Viking Pr, 1953.

Anthony, E.: The impact of mental and physical illness on family life. Am J Psychiatry, 127:2, 1970.

Arnstein, R.: Training of psychiatrists in a student mental health clinic. In Offer, D., and Masterson, J. (Eds.): Teaching and Learning Adolescent Psychiatry. Springfield, Thomas, 1971.

Auerswald, E.: Changing concepts and changing models of residential treatment. In Caplan, G., and Lebovici, S. (Eds.): Adolescence: Psychosocial Perspectives. New York, Basic, 1969.

Balser, B.: Psychotherapy of the Adolescent. New York, Int Univs Pr, 1957.

Beres, D.: Character formation. In Lorand, S., and Schneer, H. (Eds.): Adolescents: Psychoanalytic Approach to Problems and Therapy. New York, Hoeber, 1964.

Bergman, R.: Navajo peyote use: Its apparent safety. Am J Psychiatry, 128:695-699, 1971.

Berkovitz, I.: Adolescents Grow in Groups. New York, Brunner-Mazel, 1972.

Berman, S.: Psychotherapy of adolescents at clinic level. In Balser, B. (Ed.): Psychotherapy of the Adolescent. New York, Int Univs Pr, 1957.

Blos, P.: The Young Adolescent: Clinical Studies. New York, Free Pr, 1970.

Blumenthal, I. J.: Management of schizophrenia in the veteran's administration. Psychosomatics, 12:61-68, 1971.

Brown, S.: Family therapy for adolescents. Psychiatric Opinion, 7: 1970

Caplan, G.: A community mental health plan for adolescents. In Caplan, G., and Lobovici, S. (Eds.): Adolescence: Psychosocial Perspectives. New York, Basic, 1969.

Churchill, D.: Effects of success and failure. Arch Gen Psychiatry, 25:208-214, 1971.

Cline, D., and Rouser, D.: The nonphysician as primary therapist in hospital psychiatry. Am J Psychiatry, 128:4, 1971.

Cumming, J., and Cumming, E.: Ego and Milieu. New York, Atherton, 1962.

Davies, R., et al.: Confusional episodes and antidepressant medication. Am J Psychiatry, 128:127-132, 1971.

Dole, V.: Pharmacological treatment of drug addiction. Modern Medicine, February, 1972,

Erikson, E.: Identity: Youth and Crisis. New York, Norton, 1968.

Evans, J.: Personal communication.

Fenton, N.: An Introduction to Group Counseling in Correctional Service. New York, American Correctional Association, 1957.

Fish, B.: Drug use in psychiatric disorders. Am J Psychiatry, 124 (Supplement):31-36, 1968.

Fitzpatrick, J.: The therapeutic community: An alternative to methadone in the treatment of heroin addiction. Drug Therapy, 2:20-33, 1972.

French, E.: Residential Treatment for Emotionally Disturbed Young People. New York, Mental Hospitals, 1963.

Gibbens, T.: Psychiatric Studies of Borstal Lads. London, Oxford University Press, 1963.

Godenne, G.: Personal communication.

Gould, R.: Methadone reconsidered. Drug Therapy, 1:16-29, 1971.

Gralnick, A.: The family in psychotherapy. Psychiatry Quarterly Supplement, Part 2. Utica, State Hospitals Press, 1962.

Greaves, D., and Regan, P.: Psychotherapy of adolescents at intensive hospital treatment level. In Balser, B. (Ed.): Psychotherapy of the Adolescent. New York, Int Univs Pr, 1957.

Greenspoon, L., and Hedblom, P.: Amphetamine abuse. Drug Therapy, 1:16-29, 1971.

Harms, E.: Drug Addiction in Youth. New York, Pergamon, 1965.

Hendrickson, W., Holmes, D., and Waggoner, R.: Psychotherapy with hospitalized adolescents. Am J Psychiatry, 116:527-532, 1959.

Hollister, L., and Kosek, J.: Sudden death during treatment with phenothiazine derivitives. JAMA, 192:12, 1965.

Holmes, D.: The Adolescent in Psychotherapy, Boston, Little, 1969.

Jones, J.: Social Psychiatry in the Community, in Hospitals and in Prisons. Springfield, Thomas, 1962.

Jorsted, J.: Personal communication.

Josselyn, I.: Psychotherapy of adolescents at the level of private practice. In Balser, B. (Ed.): Psychotherapy of the Adolescent, New York, Int Univs Pr, 1957.

Kaplan, A.: Joint parent adolescent interview in psychotherapy. In Caplan, G., and Lebovici, S. (Eds.): Adolescence: Psychosocial Perspectives. New York, Basic, 1969.

Katz, P.: The therapy of adolescent schizophrenia. Am J Psychiatry, 127:2, 1970.

Kelly, F.: The effectiveness of survival camp training with delinquents. In forty-eighth Annual Meeting, American Orthopsychiatric Association, Washington, D.C., March 21-24, 1971.

Kenniston, K.: Youth as a stage of life. In Feinstein, A., et al. (Eds.): Adolescent Psychiatry. New York, Basic, 1971.

Koblenzer, H.: Thioridazine in management of disturbed adolescents. Corrective Psychiatry, 15:18-24, 1969.

Kraft, I.: The use of psychoactive drugs in outpatient treatment of psychiatric disorders of children. Am J Psychiatry, 124:1401-1407, 1968.

Lewis, J.: A research study of healthy families. Journal of the National Association of Private Psychiatric Hospital, 3:20-24, Spring, 1971.

Makarenko, A.: The Road of Life. (Translated by Gary, S.). London, Stanley Nott, 1936.

McWhinnie, J.: Language usage and disturbed behavior. In Caplan, G., and Lebovici, S. (Eds.): Adolescence: Psychosocial Perspectives. New York, Basic, 1969.

Mulvaney, J.: Short-term treatment of adolescents on an adult psychiatric unit. Hosp Community Psychiatry, Aug., 1970, pp. 255-257.

Muller, D.: E.C.T. in LSD psychosis: A report of three cases. Am J Psychiatry, 128:351-353, 1971.

Neff, L.: Chemicals and their effects on the adolescent ego. In Feinstein, S., Giovacchini, P., and Miller, A. (Eds.): Adolescent Psychiatry. New York, Basic, 1971, pp. 108-123.

Novick, R.: Can we design patient behavior? Journal of the National Association of Private Psychiatric Hospitals, 3:27-35, Spring, 1971.

O'Malley, K., et al.: Effect of age and sex on human drug metabolism. Br Med J, 3:607-609, 1971.

Peltz, W.: Psychotherapy of adolescents at private practice plus school practice levels. In Balser, B. (Ed.): Psychotherapy of the Adolescent. New York, Int Univs Pr, 1957.

Polak, P., and Laycob, L.: Rapid Tranquilization. Am J Psychiatry, 128:640-643, 1971.

Reidenberg, M.: Personal communication.

Rinsley, D.: Theory and practice of intensive residential treatment of adolescents. In Feinstein, S., Giovacchini, P., and Miller, G. (Eds.): Adolescent Psychiatry. New York, Basic, 1971, vol. I, pp. 479-510.

Robbins, L.: Ego psychology and the milieu at the mental hospital. Int Psychiatry Clin, 5:1. Also in Eldred, S., and Vanderpol, M. (Eds.): The Designed Therapeutic Milieu. Boston, Little, 1960.

Rubenstein, R.: Changes in psychiatric hospital organization and inter-personal conflict. In Thirty-eighth Annual Meeting, National Association Private Psychiatric Hospitals, Key Biscayne, Florida, January 25-28, 1971.

Samorajczyk, J.: Psychotherapy as meaningful parental figure with alienated adolescents. Am J Psychother, 25:110-116, 1971,

Schmideberg, M.: Personal communication.

Schoenfeld, W.: A practical approach to individual psychotherapy of the adolescents. Psychiatric Opinion, 7:1, 1970.

Searles, J.: The Therapeutic Team. Int Psychiatry Clin, 5:1. Also in Eldred, S., and Vanderpol, M. (Eds.): The Designed Therapeutic Milieu. Boston, Little, 1960.

Sklansky, M., et al.: The High School Adolescent: Understanding and Treating His Emotional Problems. New York, Ass Pr, 1969.

Stanton, A.: Introduction to psychotherapy. Int Psychiatry Clin, 5:1. Also in Eldred, S., and Vanderpol, M. (Eds.): The Designed Therapeutic Milieu, Boston, Little, 1960.

Stern, R.: Personal communication.

Taylor, M., and Levine, R.: Influence of sex of hospitalized schizophrenics on therapeutic dosage levels of neuroleptics. Dis Nerv Syst, 32:131-134, 1971.

Teichers, J.: Group psychotherapy with adolescents. Calif Med, 105:18-21, 1966.

Vanderpol, M.: The designed milieu as an extension of the psychotherapeutic process. Int Psychiatry Clin, 5:1. Also in Eldred, S., and Vanderpol, M. (Eds.): The Designed Therapeutic Milieu. Boston, Little, 1960.

Washburn, S.: Milieu interventions in the treatment of psychosis. Int Psychiatry Clin, 5:1. Also in Eldred, S., and Vanderpol, M. (Eds.): The Designed Therapeutic Milieu. Boston, Little, 1960.

Welsch, E.: Psychotherapy of the Adolescent − Discussion. In Balser, B. (Ed.): Psychotherapy of the Adolescent, New York, Int Univs Pr, 1957.

Winn, H.: Personal Communication.

Winnicott, D.: Clinical Regression Compared with Defense Organization. Int Psychiatry Clin, 5:1. Also in Eldred, S., and Vanderpol, M. (Eds.): The Designed Therapeutic Milieu. Boston, Little, 1960.
Wolf, A., et al.: Beyond the Couch. New York, Science, 1970.

Chapter V

ASPECTS OF PSYCHOTHERAPEUTIC TECHNIQUE

TECHNICAL literature dealing with the psychotherapy of adolescents has grown greatly in the recent past and is still in the process of development. While this area of treatment incorporates aspects of both adult and child psychotherapy, it is nonetheless quite separate and distinct and an entity of its own.

Important recent contributors in the field are Hendrickson, Holmes (1969), Balser, Blos (1962), Masterson (1967), Rinsley (1967), Gralnick, Glasser (1965), among a host of others. Sigmund Freud, Anna Freud, Aichorn, Reich and Deutsch were earlier psychoanalytic writers who contributed much technical as well as theoretical information about treatment of the adolescent.

Rather than present a panoramic review of the technical literature, this chapter will focus upon some key aspects of adolescent psychotherapy and attempt to provide a meaningful frame of reference for the beginning clinician.

THE CLINICAL FRAME OF REFERENCE: PSYCHODYNAMIC

The psychoanalytic literature has provided important theoretical concepts to help understand not only the adolescent phase of development, but all human behavior as well. While it is not within the scope of this book to attempt to validate or invalidate these psychoanalytic concepts, from an operational and clinical point of view, they are most helpful.

Psychic determinism, phases of psychosexual development, transference, defenses, the Oedipal struggle, identity, ego development, separation, individuation, the unconscious, orality, and dependency are all constructs that are of value in comprehending the human organism in its march from childhood dependency towards adulthood.

In general terms these concepts portray the individual growing up through discrete phases of psychological development. Successful completion of each phase is determined not only by the richness of the individual's endowments and the support derived from the family and society but also by the degree of success achieved in mastering previous phases of psychobiological development. The greater the success with one phase, the easier will be the transition throughout subsequent phases. Conversely, the more there are residual conflicts, traumas and stresses, the more difficult subsequent passage will be. Thus, childhood experiences have a direct influence upon adolescent experience.

Psychic determinism and the unconscious are notions which contend that all behavior has a cause, but the cause may not always be apparent to the individual involved; that an unconscious repository exists for the roots of much behavior and attitudes which can only be uncovered and understood by special technique and careful study.

Under certain circumstances, individuals unconsciously attempt to reestablish important childhood relationships from the past in current adult relationships, imputing to contemporary figures qualities they really do not possess. This form of perceptual distortion of current object relationships is called *transference.* The individual is simply looking for important characteristics of parental figures in current relationships. While this tendency can gratify certain infantile needs, it may produce much social stress. Comprehension of these transference distortions is an important part of adolescent treatment.

The individual's personality is a composition of all of his psychological traits and attitudes, the sum and substance of which renders him unique and with an identity all his own. The individual facets of personality are acquired in different ways, but identification with the qualities of others plays a key role in psychological development. To change certain aspects of an individual's personality is very difficult as it strikes at the very roots of his sense of self. Resistances and defenses may be construed, then, as the individual's attempt to preserve his psychological life, no matter how maladaptive or "sick" it may be. In this context, therapeutic intervention and the personality changes it produces might thus be seen as a threat to one's psychological integrity and existence and defended against on that basis. The adolescent patient will stop resisting treatment and accept change when he is convinced that he can trust the therapist not to let him down; that the therapist will replace what is lost with something better.

Adolescent Psychodynamic Psychotherapy

Psychoanalytic techniques, as developed by Freud and his followers, were designed essentially for adult patients.

Anna Freud, Klein, Mahler, and Blos, among others, pioneeered modifications in analytic technique for children and young people. Josselyn stressed the need to support the adolescent's ego continually during the course of treatment; Greenson, Holmes, Hwinn and Vanderpol noted the importance of recognizing emergent transference phenomena during therapy, as manifested by unstated expectations, special patterns of behavior, anxiety, flight from treatment, or difficulties in the terminating phase of psychotherapy. Loeb and Kremer elaborated upon the difficulties posed by both positive and negative transference.

The following vignette illustrates the difficulties posed by a negative transference situation:

Case

Sally, an attractive fifteen-year-old girl, was brought to the psychiatrist for assaultiveness to her parents. She presented all the appearances of a young tigress and had been a part of a violent street gang for some time, though her parents were well-educated, middle class people. The family dynamics consisted of a devitalized parental relationship with Sally forming a powerful coalition with her mother. While Mother felt it, Sally openly expressed her contempt for her father with four letter words. His desperate attempt to assert leadership in the family resulted in a physical brawl between father and daughter and her subsequent hospitalization.

At the outset, her hostility towards him was intense while she was establishing a positive working relationship with her male therapist. In separate sessions, her parents began to work out their marital differences and to move closer together. When they resisted Sally's attempts to manipulate and polarize them, she began to withdraw and lose interest in both of them. At the same time, her attitude towards her therapist started to change radically. Instead of the open, friendly, grinning gamine, there reemerged the tigress, negative, resistive and insulting. She vowed that she could not work with her therapist as he did not understand her; she began to absent herself from the hospital for periods of time, coming back "high" on drugs, reminiscent of her behavior when she was living at home. Both the therapist and her father were thus the same to her, exhibiting an inability to prevent this behavior. As soon as her improved behavior would warrent greater privileges, she would again go off, take drugs and return to demonstrate her anger and contempt towards her therapist. The parallel between father and therapist was complete. Once Sally was able to recreate the intense hostile father-relationship with the therapist, little could be done to salvage treatment.

Loeb points out that not all of the patient's behavior towards the therapist should be viewed as manifestations of transference. The adolescent may relate in an entirely reality-oriented manner or he may show evidences of identification with the psychotherapist. Differentiating these patterns of behavior from one another is important not only in helping the clinician understand the patient but also in framing the correct interpretations.

Other modifications of psychoanalytic technique can be effective in adolescent psychotherapy. The psychoanalytic requisite for four or five sessions per week may be inappropriate when treating young people. Initial contact on a once-a-week basis may be all a threatened adolescent can tolerate at first. Double sessions may be indicated for some young patients who are slow in getting started. The use of psychoanalytic couch can be made optional. When given a choice of either sit up or lie down at any time, the adolescent may find such options engaging and attractive. The use of the couch on this basis is relatively nonthreatening and aids in cutting through resistiveness and defensiveness. Positioning the patient's chair away from vis-a-vis with the therapist is also helpful in fostering introspection and minimizing intellectualization. No doubt, a variety of innovations and alterations of classical psychoanalytic technique, in the hands of a competent therapist, can serve to increase the effectiveness of adolescent psychotherapy.

Other Psychotherapies

Wolpe, Glasser, Berman, Schoenfeld and Levine describe other psychotherapeutic approaches, referred to as behavioral, reality, manipulative, educative, cathartic, directive, supportive and ego-oriented psychotherapies. No doubt other modes of treatment exist as well. Each of these therapeutic modalities pursues a special goal, focuses upon a specific aspect of adolescent psychopathology, or elaborates a special technique. Most acknowledge the fragility of the adolescent ego and the need to strengthen it rather than tear down its defenses.

THE THERAPEUTIC STANCE

After consideration of the form of psychotherapy, it is essential to deal with the therapist himself. Development of certain attitudes and styles of behavior enhance treatment, while other forms of behavior thwart the development of a therapeutic relationship. Samorajczyk (1971) sees the adolescent therapist as a parental figure, serving as an object for identification, education and insight. Greaves and Porter stress the importance of the clinician assuming the role of the friendly protector and even sanctioner, while Gittelsen (1942) differentiates between accepting the adolescent from his destructive behavior. Holmes sees the importance of setting firm, realistic limits for the young patient. Berman (1957) deals with the adolescent's capacity to exploit the anxieties and vulnerabilities of the therapist who in turn requires a strong self-image. He also has a need to avoid seeming authoritarian as well as a need to establish mutual trust. Development of a sense of mutuality between the therapist and the young patient is a requirement for the latter's ego growth and development.

In résumé, then, the ideal posture for the therapist to take should be informal, stimulating and friendly and at the same time, expectant of responsibility, reflection and mutual respect from the young patient. In many ways, the therapist seems to take on the role of the ideal parent.

In more profound and intense forms of therapy, the clinician must be alert to and prepared to deal with transference distortions of the therapist-patient relationship as well as a great deal of testing and manipulativeness.

PROGNOSTIC INDICATORS

Once the adolescent has become involved in treatment it may be helpful to erect realistic goals, and prognostic indicators can serve as a guideline. The following factors are consistent with a favorable outcome.

1. Sincere self-referral.
2. Acceptance of the concept of personal problems.
3. Presence of psychological pain.
4. Motivation to change.
5. Economic independence.
6. History of accomplishments.
7. Sense of responsibility.
8. The ability to form a working relationship with the therapist.
9. Acceptance of hospital rules and other limits.
10. Positive relationships to family or surrogates.

(Tamerin)

Of all of the above, perhaps the two most important determiners of therapeutic success are motivation to change and a history of positive accomplishments.

THE OPENING PHASE OF THERAPY

Engagement versus Resistiveness and Defensiveness

Special therapeutic techniques are often necessary to enlist the young patient into an active, positive therapeutic relationship. Unlike the adult, who often embarks upon treatment despite initial apprehension or ambivalence, the adolescent must develop good feelings about therapy and the person treating him or he will not stay. He may take to the treatment situation instantaneously or he may accept it only after much testing and stormy sessions. Techniques for involving the young patient vary, according to the patient's needs and the therapist's fortes.

Telephone tactics are important when therapy is about to begin. Requesting the young patient himself to call for the first appointment rather than some family member can be a wise strategem. It tells the prospective patient that the therapist regards him as sufficiently adult to make his own arrangements. It also provides the therapist with some indication of the adolescent's motivation for treatment. Indecision on the prospective patient's part during the initial phone call might be resolved by inviting him to bring a friend or anyone else of his choosing to the office for the first visit. This tactic is often both reassuring and intriguing and the companions selected can be interesting and significant. For instance, a pretty, strong-willed girl of sixteen elected to bring the boyfriend her parents disapproved of as a gesture of defiance and as a means of testing her therapist. An eighteen-year-old brought her more attractive seventeen-year-old sister on the first visit to see if the doctor would favor her sibling and ignore her as her family always did. Thus, the opportunity to select a companion helps overcome the resistance to the initial therapist-patient contact and at the same time can provide important insights.

Determination of the family role in the overall treatment plan is important and should be established at the very beginning. Mishandling of the family can easily produce misunderstanding and therapeutic failure.

The following principles may be helpful in establishing a workable treatment formula.

1. The primary therapeutic thrust should be directed toward the adolescent, and family involvement should be shaped in terms of what will facilitate treatment of the adolescent.

2. In some situations, only minimal contact with the family may be indicated, e.g. with an older or emancipated adolescent or when the family is not directly involved in the psychological

problem and is sufficiently secure to accept change in the young patient without becoming threatened.

3. Determination of the family dynamics is helpful in managing crises that may arise during the course of treatment. For instance, foreknowledge of the patient's propensity to flee in the face of stress may help the therapist to understand missed appointments; information about father's competitiveness or mother's dependency will clarify the urgent telephone complaint just when the young patient is starting to progress and change.

4. Seriously disturbed parents should be aided in understanding the degree of their emotional disturbances and its impact upon their child. The recommendation for them to obtain help follows naturally and is often well received. Their inclusion into family therapy with the adolescent or their treatment with another psychotherapist can then be discussed.

In any event, the family must be actively considered when beginning treatment of an adolescent.

The interest stimulated in the adolescent during the first visit is often crucial in determining whether or not treatment will proceed. At this time, the prospective young patient must be not only reassured but actively engaged in the interaction. Some key questions may be helpful in arousing the adolescent's curiosity, putting him at ease, and at the same time providing the therapist with important information. The following are illustrative:

Question: Your parents called and mentioned their concern about you. I'm not sure I fully understand. What do you suppose they're worried about?

Question: Is there anyone you'd like to bring with you next time?

Question: What things do you like to do the most? What things do you hate the most?

Question: I'd like to get to know you better. Can you tell me the most important things that happened to you? What happenings stand out most in your mind?

Question: Who's your best friend? Do you date? Do you have
as many friends as you'd like?

Asking the young patient to draw a picture of a person and then
compose a story about that person is a simple, valuable, and often
absorbing projective technique with younger adolescents. They
may also show interest in snacking, going for a walk, or playing
cards. Any patient who plays a musical instrument or who has a
record collection or a hobby might enjoy bringing these items to
the therapeutic session.

In the final analysis, perhaps the two most effective levers for
engaging the young patient in treatment are the therapist's interest
and imagination.

Resistance to psychotherapy is usual for adolescents. It is borne
of many factors, both conscious and unconscious. Fear, anger and
embarrassment are three important emotions with which to deal.
Schoenfeld (1970) cites the prevalence of intellectualization, and
Holmes (1969) lists denial, counterphobia, projection and manipulativeness as defenses and character traits that adolescents frequently use to resist treatment. Timing is a major factor with
which to contend and Barish (personal communication) stresses
the need to overcome resistances as quickly as possible before the
opportunity for therapy dissipates. The importance of the
therapist's reassuring, friendly position has already been noted by
Holmes and others.

Communication and Silence

Silence

Usually, the younger the patient is, the less likely he is to be
verbal and the less tolerant he is of silence. It is thus inappropriate
for the therapist to allow the same periods of silence to pass as he
would for an adult. In his mounting discomfort, the adolescent
will often find fault with treatment and the therapist. Early active
intrusion into silence is thus appropriate and may be handled in
several ways:

1. The therapist may simply ask the patient to put his thoughts
and feelings into words.

2. He may make reference to the silence and simply show his curiosity about it.

3. He may openly speculate about it and offer various speculations to the adolescent regarding the meaning of the silence. Again, anger, anxiety and embarrassment are frequent affects implicated; hallucinations may be producing the breakdown of verbal communication; the use of silence as a manipulative or testing device is also a possibility.

Patience, reassurance and active inquiry are often helpful in re-stimulating the flow of ideas. Introduction of another, less stressful theme may be helpful.

Communication

Communication is a term that is panoramic and often imprecise. Generally, if refers to an exchange between active and receptive participants sharing feelings, thoughts and behavior. Holmes notes that with adolescents, communication may be verbal, behavioral or autonomic, manifested by a variety of somatic signs.

Some critical determiners of communication with the young person are:

1. Feelings toward authority figures: Perception of the therapist as more powerful may be inhibitory.

2. Trust: The conviction that the possible risk engendered by getting close to the therapist will ultimately produce greater happiness and less pain.

3. Commonality of values: The interface for sharing similar feelings and views. The common ground where warm feelings can develop.

4. Language compatability: The use of words that are mutually understood. The lexicon of the adolescent is often dissimilar to that of the adult.

5. Involvement: Proof to the young person of the therapist's sustaining interest and commitment until ultimate resolution of his problems.

6. Logistics: No communication can ensue at the wrong place or at the wrong time; appropriateness of the setting is important as is the therapist's accessibility.

7. Defensiveness: Denial and intellectualization are two of

many habitual defenses of adolescence. They pose real barriers to communication of inner thoughts and feelings and their impact must be minimized.

8. Parents: Inappropriate involvement of or hostility from parents can easily thwart the adolescent's interest in therapy and the therapist.

Thus, communication hinges upon a variety of factors and their recognition may aid in removing obstacles to the sharing of experiences and to productive therapeutic effort.

THE MIDDLE PHASE OF THERAPY

This phase of psychotherapy is characterized by manifestations of transference and identification phenomena, appropriate involvement of the family, and the explicit definition of the patient's psychological problems.

Difficulties relate to negative transference, the adolescent propensity to act out, polarization and manipulation of involved adults and reality problems such as school pressures, vacations, and parental intervention.

Transference Phenomena

When the patient relates to the therapist as if he were a mother or father figure from an earlier epoch, the transference feelings can be intensely negative or positive. When the therapist is riding the crest of positive transference, immediate interpretation of the adolescent's perceptual distortions are not crucial and may be postponed until the first opportune moment. Negative transference phenomena, however, are different. Young people cannot long tolerate intensely negative feelings, and unless this transference is explained and understood, it can produce a rupture of the therapeutic alliance and the end of treatment.

The following therapeutic vignette is illustrative.

Case

Judy, an attractive and provocative fifteen-year-old was brought to the psychiatrist because of academic failure and minor delinquency.

Judy's mother was consumed with ambivalence regarding sexual values and Judy was similarly conflicted, with many bitter battles resulting between mother and daughter. Judy found herself in a continuous bind to comply with her mother's unconscious libertine values on the one hand and her more conscious needs for propriety. Thus despite the family secret that mother was involved in a messy affair several years before, Judy was still punished for her sexual interest and behavior.

As an inpatient, Judy tested her therapist frequently, imploring him to trust her with increased privileges and then abusing the confidence he placed in her. When returning two days later from a six-hour pass, she was asked what had happened to her. At that point, Judy flew into a rage, almost as if she were waiting to be asked and shrieked, "You're just like my mother." She had re-created a drama re-enacted many times before with her mother in which she was recriminated for her libertine behavior by a mother who was promiscuous herself. The negative transference to the therapist-mother was complete and there was very little he could do or say that was right in the view of the young patient.

From a tactical standpoint, such negativism is difficult to deal with. It may be diluted by enlisting the aid of another therapist who will either draw off some of the anger or help provide the patient with better perspective. A meeting with the parents may help the young patient understand the nature of the transference distortions and the basis of her overreaction to the therapist. In any event, resolution of negative transference is necessary to preserve treatment and is a challenging therapeutic task.

Body Image, Identifications and Identity

During this crucial phase of development, the adolescent must establish an altered and differently integrated sense of self, his identity. This entails, in part, reconciling himself to a new sexual body image and the anxiety it engenders (Kolb, 1959). In addition, he must master his bisexual propensity and establish a clear-cut sense of gender identity and gender roles (Gardiner, 1959). The roots of this identity sense are laid down well before the onset of puberty. A rudimentary body image and sense of self is established early in infancy with the development of hand-mouth coordination (Hoffer, 1949; Gessel and Ilg, 1942).

During adolescence, sexuality plays an important role in the establishment of a sense of self. Much behavior and many feelings stem from basic perceptions that one is male or female. Preoccupation with such secondary sex characteristics as hair, musculature and breasts provide ample testimony to the close relationship between one's sense of gender and one's sense of self at this phase.

The obligation to meet the challenge of identity and the development of new body attitudes in adolescence generates much anxiety and defensiveness (Erikson, 1950; Gardner, 1959). Withdrawal, the denial of impulses, over-control, narcissism or other psychological defenses may become manifest in the effort to cope with new drives and to establish an adult identity. At this stage, the adolescent is fragile, vulnerable and easily hurt (Kahne, 1971).

If identity is the sense of self and the experience of wholeness (Erikson, 1950), identification refers to a process of overcoming one's inherent bisexual tendency and achieving a sense of one's own gender by incorporating ideas, attitudes and roles from the parent of the same sex, or his surrogate. It also includes learning about maleness and femaleness from the parent of the opposite sex by contrast (Gardner, 1959).

Developing a clear gender identity is often an important part of the work of the adolescent's psychotherapy and getting close to or identifying with the psychotherapist facilitates the process greatly (Farnsworth, 1966). Not only does the young patient emulate some of the real characteristics of the accepted therapist (Josselyn, 1957), but also some of the fantasized characteristics of the idealized infantile parent (Kubie, 1945). The intense amount of emotional energy bestowed upon the clinician is great, and much learning, emotional growth and sound psychological development can occur by this process of identification. But this process must serve the function of ego development. The seasoned therapist should not need the gratification of being emulated by the temporarily dependent young patient nor misunderstand it or exploit it. It is merely a necessary transitory phase of treatment. Success in this endeavor on the part of the young patient should be gratification enough.

Perhaps the best means of fostering a conducive climate for growth-promoting identifications is by means of the working relationship in which the therapist's constancy, kindness and his capacity to interpret reality play major roles (See "Therapeutic Stance"). The therapist's personal values, ego strength and his own identificational certainty are also of crucial importance.

The Management of Acting Out, Polarization and Manipulativeness

Acting out is the conscious or unconscious translation of psychological stress and conflict into destructive behavior. The following case vignette is illustrative:

Case

After a period of time, Trudy responded well enough to inpatient care to be considered for discharge. She had a long history of delinquent behavior both in and out of the hospital, but the staff felt that she had grown enough to be discharged from the hospital. On the eve of a family conference to discuss Trudy's homecoming, she absconded from the hospital, only to return several days later "high" on a variety of drugs. Once again, she dramatized her feelings by translating them into a destructive act. Only later on, and with much inducement, was she able to verbalize the feelings behind the flight: that she could never again live with her parents and she expressed it in a way she knew best. Trudy was impulsive and action-oriented, and the interposition of a thought between a feeling and an action was alien to her.

The therapeutic task with the acting-out adolescent, then, is to convert destructive impulses to reflective forethought and thereby afford the young patient options and choices of behavior for the first time (Josselyn, 1957). When the individual can learn to think before taking an action, he can weigh the positive and negative aspects of such an action. His choice can be, then, in terms of what is best for him in the long run. For the immediate action under consideration, the choice can be "yes" or "no" where no choice existed before. Teaching the adolescent to think before acting is fundamental in the psychotherapy of acting-out.

The establishment of firm limits, consonant with reality, is another important part of the treatment of acting-out. Often an inpatient setting and a therapeutic milieu are essential in order to implement this limit-setting procedure (Berman, 1957).

Polarization and manipulativeness are adolescent maneuvers, the functions of which are to nullify adult authority and ultimately produce autonomy. Yet, this is a mutually desirable goal for both the adolescent and the therapist and an integral aspect of psychological maturity. But with autonomy must come a sense of responsibility and a constructive orientation. Once the therapist and the young patient can agree upon these ultimate goals, they can then become allies rather than adversaries locked in a power struggle.

On an operational level the adolescent's attempts to polarize parents, hospital staff and others in positions of authority can produce havoc in a treatment program. Slip-ups in communication, even temporary ones, can result in misunderstanding, factionalism, and even termination of treatment. In the short run, the adolescent gains a misguided sense of power and omnipotence even though he has been instrumental in wrecking a program that would have resulted in his ultimate betterment.

The tendency to polarize and manipulate is ubiquitous and not necessarily pathological, and a spirit of cooperativeness and open communication can effectively contain these maneuvers. Parents, hospital personnel and therapists must be in agreement with regards to therapeutic goals, limits to behavior and the *modus operandi*. The adolescent, testing his world for limits and detecting solidarity and unanimity, becomes greatly reassured and turns away from these defensive and often destructive tactics.

Problems of Authority

The degree of resentment and mistrust an adolescent feels and expresses towards authority figures is variable and a function of the patient, the therapist and the milieu. With the compliant, submissive patient it is superficially minimal, while with the adolescent in open rebellion it may be a major problem of treatment. The particular image that the therapist projects is often a factor determining whether or not a power struggle develops. The value system and hierarchy established in an inpatient setting can profoundly influence youthful rebelliousness.

One therapeutic approach to the management of this problem focuses upon the observation that the more one is dependent, irresponsible and out of personal control, the more one is prone to be controlled by others. Since the object of therapy is to help the young person achieve a position of self-reliance and autonomy, then both the adolescent and the therapist can be allied in developing the necessary skills as quickly as possible.

In dealing with problems of authority, it is also helpful to differentiate between the authority of power, which may produce much adolescent antagonism, and the authority of knowledge, which often evokes in him feelings of admiration. Very frequently, the young patient himself possesses expertise in a particular area and can be acknowledged as the authority by all concerned. He may be induced to teach his skill to others or give them a demonstration; he may use his fund of knowledge as a basis for barter or popularity. In any event, his knowledge or skill can be converted into source of heightened self-esteem and "status."

Thus, the problem of authority can be converted into an exercise in personal responsibility and a springboard to a more positive self-image rather than a source of humiliation and rebellion.

THE FINAL PHASE

Premature Termination

Psychotherapy with the adolescent often fails to run full course, being interrupted prematurely for a variety of reasons. However, failure to bring the adolescent patient to a point of mutually agreed-upon termination does not necessarily indicate therapeutic failure. In a follow-up study of discharged adolescent inpatients hospitalized for periods as brief as twenty one days, considerable changes in their life styles were notable. These included resumption of schooling or enrollment in a vocational training program, salutary changes in their domicile, improved social life, improved subjective feelings, and fewer altercations with the law (Follow-Up Study, Northwestern Mental Health Center, unpublished).

Oftentimes, patients hospitalized for the second time become asymptomatic relatively rapidly and resume their psychotherapeutic efforts from where they left off during the last hospital stay. In some cases, it seems as if the patient had never been away.

Thus, a period of treatment not going to completion may still be a very valuable experience for the young patient.

Transference and Dependency

The kind of full-blown transference neurosis noted in the psychoanalysis of certain adults usually does not develop with adolescents in psychotherapy. Less tightly organized transference phenomena, on the other hand, consisting of inappropriate, strong emotional attachments, feelings of dependency, or intensely negative and rebellious attitudes, are not unusual. Other forms of transference stereotypes are also noted and include manifestations of excessive and inappropriate fear and the expectation of rejection and disapproval.

Positive transference phenomena, somewhat resembling hero worship, can be an extremely important force for the resumption of ego growth and emotional development. After treatment is terminated, a residuum of warm feelings towards the therapist often remain, and are benign.

The management of negative transference presents a difficult therapeutic task. Resolution of his anger and rebelliousness during the course of psychotherapy, with the concomitant development of a sense of personal authority, integrity and responsibility can be a greatly beneficial learning experience to the adolescent.

A successful therapeutic course leads to the resumption of normal development and re-entrance into the mainstream of adolescent life. The resulting decreased dependency on the therapist, associated with a burgeoning of outside interests and peer relationships, tends to diminish transference phenomena.

Residual problems of dependency and negative transference may persist, however, and should not be left unattended. If they should persist at the point of termination of therapy, it is important that the young patient is made aware of this state of feelings, possible genetic reasons for them as well as their possible consequences in the future. Psychotherapy at some time in the future can be recommended should these unresolved problems prove burdensome.

INDICES OF PROGRESS

The following indices denote progress made in psychotherapy:
1. Increased outside interests.
2. Increased peer relationships, both quantitively and qualitatively.
3. Improved family relations.
4. Improved self-concept.
5. Improved academic function.
6. Diminution of symptoms (Berman, 1957).

True progress and real ego growth should be differentiated from pseudoprogress where the patient loses his symptoms and flees from treatment. This "flight into health" is not a true expression of growth and progress but is rather a function of fear and flight from deeper personality problems that are about to be uncovered in psychotherapy.

In such situations, anxiety is the key affect and should be interpreted to the patient along with the reasons for its emergence. Should the patient insist upon leaving treatment anyway, the therapist may politely disagree with the patient's evaluation and indicate that the door is always open for the resumption of therapy at another time.

Many young people do interrupt their treatment temporarily and resume it at a later date so long as they feel that it's all right to do so.

BIBLIOGRAPHY

Barish, J.: Personal communication.
Berman, S.: Psychotherapy of Adolescents at Clinic Level. New York, University Press, 1957.
Blos, P.: On Adolescence. Glencoe, The Free Press, 1962.

Erikson, E.: Childhood and Society. New York, Norton, 1950.

Erikson, E.: Insight and Responsibility. New York, Norton, 1964.

Farnsworth, D.: Psychiatric Education and the Young Adult. Springfield, Thomas, 1966.

Gardner, G.: Psychiatric problems of adolescence. In Ariette, A. (Ed.): American Handbook of Psychiatry. New York, Basic, 1959, vol. I, pp. 870-895.

Gesell, A., and Ilg, F.: Infant and Child in the Culture of Today. New York, Harper, 1942.

Gittelson, M.: Direct psychotherapy in adolescence. Am J Orthopsychiatry, 12:1-25, 1942.

Glasser, W.: Reality Therapy. New York, Harper, 1965.

Greaves, D., and Regan, P.: Psychotherapy of adolescents at intensive hospital treatment level. In Balser, B. (Ed.): Psychotherapy of the Adolescent. New York, Int Univs Pr, 1957.

Hoffer, W.: Mouth, hand and ego interaction. In The Psychoanalytic Study of the Child. New York, Int Univs Pr, 1949, vol. III, pp. 49-56.

Holmes, D.: The Adolescent in Psychotherapy. Boston, Little, 1969.

Josselyn, I.: Psychotherapy at the level of private practice. In Balser B. (Ed.): Psychotherapy of the Adolescent. New York, Int Univs Pr, 1957.

Kahne, M.: Education of psychiatrists for college practice. In Offer, D. and Masterson, J. (Eds.): Teaching and Learning Adolescent Psychiatry. Springfield, Thomas, 1971.

Kolb, L.: Disturbances in body image. In Arietti, S. (Ed.): The American Handbook of Psychiatry. New York, Basic, 1959, vol. I, pp. 325-347.

Kubie, L.: Motivation and rehabilitation. Psychiatry, 8:69-78, 1945.

Levine, M.: Principles of psychiatric treatment. In Alexander, F., and Ross, H. (Eds.): Dynamic Psychiatry, Chicago, Chicago Univ. Press, 1952.

Mahler, M.: On Human Symbiosis and the Vicissitudes on Individuation. New York, Int Univs Pr, 1968.

Masterson, J.: The Psychiatric Dilemma of Adolescence. Boston. Little, 1967.

Meade, M.: Coming of Age in Samoa. New York, The American Library, 1950.

Peltz, W.: Psychotherapy of adolescents at private practice plus school practice levels. In Balser, B. (Ed.): Psychotherapy of The Adolescent. New York, Int Univs Pr, 1957.

Rinsley, D.: The adolescent in residential treatment: Some critical reflections. Adolescence, 2:83-95, 1967.

Samorajezyk, J.: Psychotherapist as Meaningful Parental Figure with Alienated Adolescents. Am J Psychotherapy, 25:110-116, 1971.

Schonfeld, W.: A practical approach to individual psychotherapy of the adolescent. Psychiatric Opinion, 7:1-   , 1970.

CHAPTER VI

EDUCATION, VOCATION
AND ADAPTATION

INTRODUCTION

FROM a psychological standpoint, transition from adolescence to adulthood is a difficult process and a signal event in the life of a young person. Different cultures respond to this transition with differing degrees of recognition and support.

In the advanced technical society that is America today, achievement of adult status is, to a large degree, contingent upon the ability to develop a suitable work role and achieve economic independence. These tasks require increasing preparation and training and thereby impose an expanding burden upon youth.

Adaptational success and the adoption of a societally sanctioned life's work is influenced by many factors. Cultural values and stability play an important role as do subcultural influences, family dynamics and individual psychology.

With regard to the American culture, our expanding technocracy and quest for a position of world primacy through technical achievement places great educational demands upon our young people. School curriculae are constantly upgraded to keep step with scientific advances and the information explosion. But as our society seeks more from its youth educationally, it does not always provide the necessary supports.

As costs of education and training go up, financial help must rise proportionately. Yet no uniform program of economic aid for students exists. Changing national priorities, which profoundly affect job markets and careers, must be communicated somehow to young people to aid them in career planning. Yet there is a paucity of such communication. Coordinating agencies, in close contact with training facilities, private industry and government economic planning agencies, should be developed for the purpose of guiding youth into appropriate channels of productivity. Much of the unemployment, educational disruption and frustration produced by economic shifts in the past could thereby be diminished (Herford, 1969).

The pluralistic American society described by Douglas is composed of a number of subcultures, each of which can influence its youth differently. In the recent past a youth culture has developed which has profoundly influenced adolescent transition. It has championed values that, in many ways, run counter to the central ethic of the American society. As a result, many young people have rejected such basic concepts as industriousness, marriage and the family, and formal education, and have joined the ranks of the alienated and noncommitted.

The family plays an important role in adolescent transition. In Rousselet's (1969) study of academic achievement, family interest in the student's pursuits was an important determiner of his success. Conversely, students of disinterested parents showed the poorer scholastic records.

Psychological factors are also important. The more an adolescent is free of mental problems the better he will perform academically and the less stressful will be his passage through this difficult period of development (Herford, 1969).

Analysis of the "dropout" provides interesting insight into the multiple forces that produce this educational and cultural default among the ranks of so many young people.

At the college level, current figures indicate a 40 percent dropout rate among incoming freshmen, occurring mostly at state universities and among students coming from rural areas. While disenchantment with the inadequacies and inconsistencies of the particular school or social system were often the stated reasons for leaving school, anger and frustration, derived from psychological rather than sociological sources, were often the key factors. In addition, parental conflict, poor high school grades, low college scores, and inappropriate college placement were also important determiners (Farnsworth, 1966).

Factors often associated with the high school dropout were chronic academic failure, poverty, family instability and personal problems (Sklansky).

Psychiatrically, students leaving school prematurely may present a broad spectrum of emotional illnesses which include the neuroses and psychosomatic diseases as well as schizophrenia and the drug-induced psychoses.

From a psychodynamic standpoint, academic failure in the presence of chronic family discord often represents retaliation on the student's part towards one or both parents, a renunciation of vicarious parental ambitions, or guilt over an exaggerated sense of competitiveness towards a parent (Marcus, 1969).

Thus, dropping out of school can be a reflection of many sociological and psychological factors. While such an act may appear, on the surface, as a deliberate renunciation of questionable academic pursuits, it may well be a reflection of psychological breakdown and default instead.

SPECIAL ADAPTATIONAL PROBLEMS OF EMOTIONALLY DISTURBED YOUTH

The emotionally disturbed adolescent, frequently no more than marginally adjusted in school, often succumbs to increasing educational pressures and falls by the academic wayside (Marcus, 1969).

The psychologically ill youth fails academically for a number of reasons:
1. Inappropriateness of traditional modes of teaching
2. Heightened adolescent rebelliousness
3. Cumulative educational deficit
4. The emotional illness per se

Inappropriateness of Traditional Modes of Teaching

Attempting to remotivate a student who has lost interest in learning by virtue of chronic failure is difficult. Two technical problems further complicate this task: the traditional use of time and traditional curriculae.

In the last decade the entire fabric of the educational system has been undergoing intense scrutiny and profound change (Gordon, 1966), and inspection of the educational approach to the disturbed adolescent is important.

With regard to time blocks, the practice of packaging information in six-month parcels, called semesters, has little relevance to the disturbed, bored, negativistic adolescent short on attention. His interest often runs in terms of minutes rather than months.

The relevance of curriculae has already been challenged, but usually on sociological grounds (Eckstein, 1969). The applicability of traditional courses to the teaching of emotionally disturbed youngsters should be questioned as well. Frequently courses and their contents are geared to the requirements of state boards of education and college entrance rather than to the special needs of special students. The essential ingredient in all such courses should be the capacity to generate interest and enthusiasm where boredom and negativism prevailed, and this requires much creativity and flexibility on the part of educators.

Heightened Adolescent Rebelliousness

To question authority is one of the essential characteristics of adolescence and an important ingredient in student protest. Rightly or wrongly, students frequently focus upon the educational system and its teachers as perpetrators of wrongdoing and label them authoritarian, irrelevant and hypocritical. This rebelliousness is ubiquitous (A. Freud, 1969), has always existed in different guises, and must be understood by educators for what it is: one form of the adolescent quest for separation, individuation, recognition and eventual parity. Thus, a challenge to the establishment is to be expected and even welcomed, but when it becomes exaggerated or destructive, it may be quite pathological (Nixon, 1964). This hostile destructiveness often proves a formidable barrier to group learning or group process of any form.

Cumulative Educational Deficit

A cumulative educational deficit presupposes that an insufficient learning experience at one grade level renders the task of succeeding at the next grade level more difficult; that this informational handicap is often chronic and cumulative, eventually producing an insurmountable deficit of skills and critical information, ending in ultimate academic failure. The emotionally disturbed adolescent, frequently unable to learn, suffering a cumulative educational deficit and embittered by a prolonged negative learning experience, frequently resists traditional learning programs (Copeland, 1974).

The Emotional Illness Per Se

Three educational problems associated with emotional disturbance are those of:
1. Learning disability
2. Thinking disorder
3. The exaggerated need for immediate gratification.

Learning Disability

The incapacity to learn by virtue of psychological illness is a phenomenon that is complex and multifaceted. This intellectual incapacitation may be a reflection of crippling anxiety, preoccupation with conflictual themes rather than the didactic material at hand, contamination of the learning experience with conflicts over success and failure, or a sense of basic defeatism and hopelessness borne of repeated failure. These mechanisms are but a few of those associated with learning disability.

Thinking Disorders

The thinking process of the psychotic adolescent is qualitatively and quantitatively different from that of the nonpsychotic and often crowds out the more normative, reality-oriented, problem solving, rational thinking necessary for traditional learning. The schizophrenic may be over-literal or concretistic and unable to think in abstract terms; he may be neologistic, using words in a personal, symbolic way, thereby stripping them of their universality and communicational value; he may be so exquisitely paranoid that no one may be perceived without alarm or anger. He may be so confused and toxic from drugs or so withdrawn or intellectually impoverished that any hope of engaging him in orthodox educational endeavors is usually quite fruitless. The floridly psychotic adolescent is not a candidate for learning traditional subjects in traditional ways.

The Heightened Need for Immediate Gratification

Sigmund Freud noted that an important determiner of maturity was the ability to postpone gratification until some time in the future, if necessary. The need for immediate pleasure, inherent in children, often noted in adolescents, and exaggerated in disturbed youth, often interferes with learning. In the traditional educational model, it is averred that hard and proficient work, sustained over a sufficient period of time, will result in reward and pleasure. How alien is this conception to many young people whose goals are immediate relief from feelings of failure and tension, and the experience of pleasure "right now"? Getting "high" is the pleasure of the moment with little or no interest in, or understanding of, tomorrow (Copeland, 1974).

Other adaptational problems befalling the emotionally disturbed adolescent are those of repeated hospitalizations, poor work adjustment, and inadequate vocational guidance. Multiple hospitalizations occurring at the crucial developmental phase of adolescence is highly disruptive, can occur fairly frequently (Lucero and Vail, 1970), and is associated with a generally poor subsequent social adjustment (Rosen, et al., 1971). Work instability is also a problem of young patients discharged from mental hospitals, (Sturm and Lipton, 1970). The incapacity to stick to one job and advance in it was correlated with such factors as the amount of residual psychopathology at the time of discharge, the amount of positive accomplishments prior to hospitalization, and marital status (Hall, et al., 1966).

Thus, young people with psychiatric disturbances have a heightened need for special vocational preparation and counselling. Yet little help of this nature is available (McFarlane, 1969).

PROPOSED SOLUTIONS TO THE PROBLEM
OF ADOLESCENT ADAPTATIONAL ARREST

It has become increasingly apparent that adequate treatment of psychologically disturbed youth requires more than the removal of psychopathological symptoms. The young person suffering from mental illness is also a victim of impaired learning, an arrest in emotional and psychological development, and a variety of adaptational difficulties. Adequate care, therefore, must go beyond symptom abatement and be broadened to include efforts to foster resumption of developmental and adaptational pursuits. This would include training in social skills, human relationships, positive self-image, self-reliance and work skills.

Some special educational and vocational programs have been proposed or already developed in this connection.

The following approaches to the task of facilitating adolescent transition are illustrative.

The Development of Coordinating Agencies

The establishment of special coordinating organizations to aid young people in making career choices represents a relatively new and interesting approach to the problem of vocational guidance (Herford, 1969). Prototypes of such agencies already exist in several European countries. Their function is to coordinate the activities of schools and training centers with labor unions, the business sector, and the different governmental agencies, thereby assuring maximum communication and guidance for young people soon to enter the job market (Marcus, 1969). Further development of such organizations could remove much of the stress and uncertainty inherent in growing up and the achievement of a suitable productive adult role.

The Development of Urban Programs

During the last decade, a variety of programs has been developed to aid young people of the inner city. The neighborhood Youth Corps is one example. It was established under the Economic Opportunity Act of 1964 and was designed to provide job training for young people age sixteen to twenty-one coming from low income families. The candidates were often dropouts or poor students, and placement focused upon jobs in hospitals and outdoor construction projects. Many programs were developed through the neighborhood Youth Corps.

The Job Corps, which began in 1965, also concerned itself with the vocational problems of dropouts. It experimented with new teaching methods and materials in its rehabilitative efforts, and placed a high premium upon enrichment experiences. It was designed to promote self-confidence and intellectual curiosity (Wilson and Lyons, 1961).

The Reverend Leon Sullivan's Office of Economic Opportunity (O.E.O.) is an organization that approaches the problem of rehabilitation of ghetto youth via self-help, vocational programs and with apparent success.

The Development of Hospital Programs

An ever-increasing number of training programs for hospitalized young people are being developed. They offer a variety of services, ranging from tutorial help to the availability of fully accredited high school programs; from vocational guidance to training schools and placement services.

Goldburgh and Rotman (1970) note the importance of continued academic activity in a hospital setting, but such educational activity must be modified to fit the special needs of the student-patients and the hospital milieu. Several factors need to be considered in this context:

Length of Stay

The rehabilitative approach to the young person in crisis and hospitalized for a short period has needs that are quite different from the adolescent confined to a residential setting for a period of months or years. Only in such a long-term setting can more formal educational and vocational programs be instituted.

Academic or Work Status

Young patients enrolled in a school or working at the time of admission will need help in order to maintain their positions while hospitalized. Appropriate liaison can be helpful in those situations where knowledge of mental illness by the authorities would not stigmatize the young person. Tutorial help is also valuable in helping the student keep abreast in these short-term situations.

On the other hand, adolescents who have discontinued their education and who have held no steady jobs must be evaluated in terms of their potential for additional training and education. Assessment of motivation as well as psychological and vocational potentials is indicated in such situations.

Mental Status

The young psychotic patient's capacity to think realistically and learn is naturally impaired by his illness. On the other hand, he may show interest in certain conflict-free areas which can be encouraged and which can serve as the basis for important therapeutic interaction. The young psychotic girl's interest in dolls may prove to be the basis of a learning experience about motherhood and birth, just as the boy's interest in a small model car may be the springboard for learning about many facets of auto mechanics. These interests have been observed even during the most florid phases of psychosis.

Motivation

Young patients who have dropped out of school or work or who have experienced only failure are often intensely negative about learning or training of any kind. Their attitudes are often defeatist and rejecting. Only when they can be intellectually stimulated and absorbed in a subject will they participate, and only the most skilled and gifted teachers can motivate such young people this way. Often an informed, creative, success-oriented learning experience can be helpful in rekindling enthusiasm and curiosity and in guiding the "dropout" back into developmental pursuits.

While broader goals of education and training are appropriate for the long-term adolescent inpatient, programs for acutely disturbed young people would have more modest objectives:

1. To foster learning experiences in psychotic patients in an effort to promulgate reality-oriented, secondary process thinking.

2. To provide enrolled students with tutorial help when indicated.

3. To provide young dropouts with a successful and intellectually stimulating work experience and thereby rekindle interest in further development.

4. To teach social skills via the group experience of learning (Copeland, 1974).

Two illustrations of long-term residential training programs are those of the Institute of the Pennsylvania Hospital in Philadelphia which has developed a fully accredited high school both for inpatients and outpatients, and Elwyn Institute also in Pennsylvania, which operates its own licensed trade school

Hillside Hospital in New York has a prevocational service for hospitalized young adults which prepares them for suitable trades, while at the same time their corollary psychotherapy focuses upon the psychological problems that have produced academic and vocational failure in the past (Diasio and Jones, 1970).

Dingleton Hospital in Scotland, where Maxwell Jones developed the therapeutic community, provides an active job counseling and placement service for its discharged patients (personal communication).

Thus, many residential centers for disturbed young people take cognizance of the need for teaching and training as part of an overall therapeutic approach and have developed a variety of programs and techniques appropos.

Development of College Programs

The college work-study program constitutes an approach designed to aid the college student in selecting a career. The curriculum is extended from four to five years, with work periods interspersed throughout to provide the student ample opportunity to gain experience in fields of possible interest. Now, thirty-eight colleges participate in work-study programs since the University of Cincinnati pioneered this concept in 1906 (Marcus, 1969).

The officially-sanctioned academic withdrawal for students

facing indecision and stress constitutes a supportive development of note on the part of institutions of higher learning. Whereas before, readmission to college was difficult after dropping out of school, a more liberal policy towards temporary withdrawal facilitates resumption of education at a later date when the student is ready.

Development of Programs in Correctional Facilities

As part of an overall Civil Rights movement, focus has again been drawn to the inequities in the penal system. Consequently, forces promulgating reform and rehabilitation have been instrumental in expanding intramural educational and vocational training programs. In many prisons, courses are offered for credit at the high school and even college level. In one institution, a two hundred hour program of formal instruction was provided to a group of prisoners nearing parole and, in a follow-up study, their recedivism rate was half that of a control group not receiving such instruction (Psychiatric News, 1971). Many such studies are indicated to determine the extent to which prisoners, especially the younger ones, are potentially trainable and salvageable.

Thus, acknowledgement of youth's needs for support and guidance through his difficult years of transition comes from many contexts. More work needs to be done, especially for the adolescent who is mentally ill.

BIBLIOGRAPHY

Babigian, A., et al.: Diagnostic consistency and change in a follow-up study of 1215 patients. Am J Psychiatry, 121:   , 1965.

Bill, A.: Social clubs help prevent readmission. Hosp Community Psychiatry, 25:161-162, 1970.

Conant, J.: Are schools getting better?. U.S. News and World Report 1967.

Copeland, A.: An interim educational program for hospitalized adolescents. To be published in Annals of Adolescent Psychiatry, Vol. III, 1974.

Diasio, K., and Jones, M.: Prevocational services for young adult psychiatric patients. Hosp Community Psychiatry, 21:217-220, 1970.

Douglas, J.: Youth in turmoil. Public Health Services Publication No. 2058, U.S. Govt Printing Office, Washington, D.C.

Eckstein, R.: Review of Bruno Betelheim's "The Children of the Dream." Psychiatry and Social Science Review, 3:8, 1969.

Farnsworth, D.: Psychiatry Education and the Young Adult. Springfield, Thomas, 1966.

Freud, A.: Adolescence as a developmental disturbance. In Caplan, G., and Lebovici, S. (Eds.): Adolescence: Psychosocial Perspectives. New York, Basic, 1969.

Goldburgh, S., and Rotman, C.: Problems in teaching hospitalized adolescents. Hosp Community Psychiatry, 21:286-289, 1970.

Gordon, I.: The Task of the Teacher Studying the Child in School. New York, Wiley, 1966,

Hall, J., et al.: Employment problems of schizophrenic patients. Am J Psychiatry, 123:5, 1966.

Hammer, S., Campbell, V., and Wolley, J.: Treating adolescent obesity. Clin Pediat, (Phila), 10:46-52, 1971.

Hasburger, A.: Educational considerations in discharging juveniles. Hosp Community Psychiatry, 21:401-402, 1970.

Herford, N.: School to work. In Caplan, G., and Lebovici, S. (Eds.): Adolescence: Psychosocial Perspectives. New York, Basic, 1969.

Hospital and Community Psychiatry. 21:195-204, 1970.

Jones, D.: Dingleton Hospital. personal communication.

Lucero, R., and Vail, D.: A comparison of three types of residential treatment programs for adolescents. Hosp Community Psychiatry, 21:181-183, 1970.

Lurie, A., and Roy, H.: Family centered after-care for young adults. Hosp Community Psychiatry, 21:35-36, 1970.

Marcus, J.: From school to work: Certain aspects of psychosocial interaction. In Caplan, G., and Lebovici, S. (Eds.): Adolescence: Psychosocial Perspectives. New York, Basic, 1969.

McFarlane, B.: The socialization of boys and girls at school and work: A Canadian study. In Caplan, G., and Lebovici, S. (Eds.): Adolescence: Psychosocial Perspectives. New York, Basic, 1969.

Nixon, R.: Psychological normalcy in the years of youth. Teachers College Record, 66:1, 1964.

Psychiatric News: "New reeducation project said to lower recidivism," Jan 10, 1971.

Psychiatric News: "Criminal patients disruptive in civil hospitals," Aug 4, 1971.

Rosen, B., et al.: Prediction of rehospitalization. J Nerv Ment Diseases, 152:17-22, 1971.

Rousselet, J.: The perception by adolescents of the role of parents in guidance and job choice. In Caplan, G., and Lebovici, S. (Eds.): Adolescence: Psychosocial Perspectives. New York, Basic, 1969.

Sturm, I., and Lipton, H.: Preparing former patients for jobs. Hosp Community Psychiatry, 21:48, 1970.

Wilson, J., and Lyons, E.: Work Study College Programs: Appraisal and Report of the Study of Cooperative Education. New York, Harper, 1961.

INDEX

A

Ability to enjoy sex, 12
"Abnormal," cultural definition, 6
Academic failure, reasons, 125
Accidents, psychogenic, 46
Acting out propensity, 10
Acting out and psychotherapy, 117
Active view of life, 12
Acute organic brain syndrome, 57
Acute, presenting problems in treatment, 78
Adaptational arrest, solutions, 128-135
   college programs, 132
   coordinating programs, 129
   correctional facility programs, 133
   hospital programs, 130-132
   urban programs, 129
Adaptational problems of mentally ill, 11, 125
Adjunctive Therapy, 94-96
Adjustment reaction of adolescence, 30-31
Adolescence, psychological characteristics, 7
Adolescent-initiated treatment contract, 79-80
Adolescent pregnancy forms, 49
Adolescent treatment, basic concepts of, 84
Adolescent value system and normality, 7
Affective disturbances, 21, 31-36
Affects, characteristics, 10
Alienation disturbance, 63-64
Amotivational syndrome, 56, 79
Amphetamines, 58
Anorexia nervosa, 29, 66-67
Antidepressants, 98
Anxiety disturbance, 34
   physiological manifestations, 34

Assessment of treatment motivation, 79
Asthma, 68
Authority problems in psychotherapy, 118

B

Bad trip, 57
Barbiturates, 59
Basic concepts of psychopathology, 20-21
Basic concepts of treatment, 84
Basic identity disturbance, 21, 24-25
Behavior, characteristic of adolescence, 10
Behavior disturbances, 36-62
Behavior, inhibition of, 10
Body image and psychotherapy, 115-117

C

Cannabis sativa, 55-56
Characteristics, psychological, 7, 8-10
Chronic presenting problems, 78
Classification of drug users, 53-55
Classification of psychopathology, 21
Clinician's intuition and clinical evaluation, 12
Cocaine, 58
College programs and adaptation, 132
Communication, 113-114
   in psychotherapy, 112
Conformism, 9
Continuum of care, 85
Coordination agencies and adaptation, 129
Correctional facilities and treatment, 87
Correctional facility programs, 133
Cultural adaptation
   judgements, 5
   modes, 5

137